Overview-M

D0207018

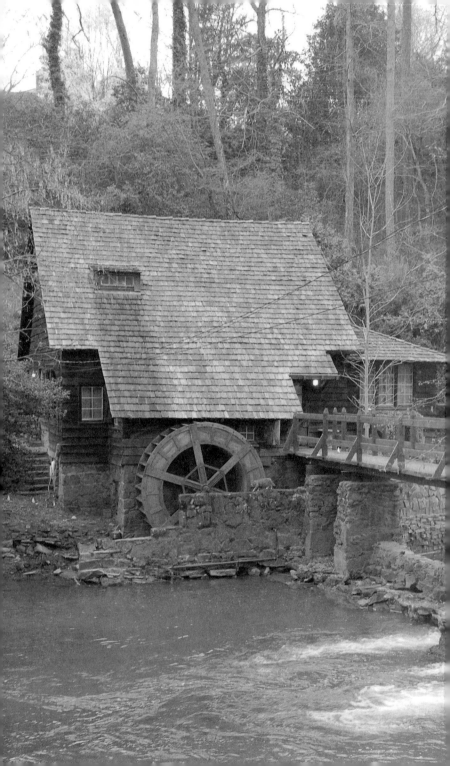

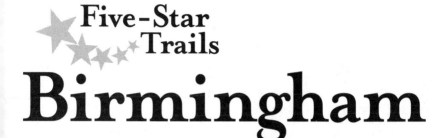

Five-Star Trails

Trails

Birmingham

Your Guide to the Area's Most Beautiful Hikes

Thomas Spencer

MENASHA RIDGE PRESS
menasharidge.com

Five-Star Trails: Birmingham
Your Guide to the Area's Most Beautiful Hikes

Copyright © 2014 by Thomas Spencer
All rights reserved
Published by Menasha Ridge Press
Distributed by Publishers Group West
Printed in the United States of America
First edition, first printing

Project editor: Ritchey Halphen
Cover design and cartography: Scott McGrew
Text design: Annie Long
Cover and interior photos: Thomas Spencer
Copyeditor: Kate McWhorter Johnson
Proofreader: John Michael Arnaud
Indexer: Rich Carlson

Frontispiece: The Old Mill on Shades Creek, Mountain Brook *(see Hike 6)*

Cataloging-in-Publication data for this book is available from the Library of Congress.

 MENASHA RIDGE PRESS
An imprint of Keen Communications, LLC
PO Box 43673
Birmingham, AL 35243
menasharidgepress.com

DISCLAIMER

This book is meant only as a guide to select trails in and around Birmingham, Alabama, and does not guarantee hiker safety in any way—you hike at your own risk. Neither Menasha Ridge Press nor Thomas Spencer is liable for property loss or damage, personal injury, or death that may result from accessing or hiking the trails described in this guide. Be especially cautious when walking in potentially hazardous terrains with, for example, steep inclines or drop-offs. Do not attempt to explore terrain that may be beyond your abilities. Please read carefully the introduction to this book, as well as safety information from other sources. Familiarize yourself with current weather reports and maps of the area you plan to visit (in addition to the maps provided in this guidebook). Be cognizant of park regulations, and always follow them. While every effort has been made to ensure the accuracy of the information in this guidebook, land and road conditions, phone numbers and websites, and other information are subject to change.

Contents

Dedication

*I dedicate this book to our collective effort to preserve,
protect, and improve access to this unique patch of the
planet we've been blessed with.*

Acknowledgments

I AM GRATEFUL FOR THE ASSISTANCE of the staff and volunteers at the various federal, state, and local parks and preserves who aided me in compiling the information in this book and who work daily to support our enjoyment of these places.

I thank Scot Duncan, Jim Lacefield, and Marjorie White, who have produced great reference books I depended on and who rendered direct assistance that helped me put this book together. Information about their books and others is included in Appendix A (page 284).

Red Mountain Park Ranger Eric McFerrin helped me understand the park's mining history. Patrick Daniel and Timothy Lee helped me get the lay of the land on Ruffner Mountain. Randy McDaniel, a friend and landscape architect, helped me identify flowers and vegetation. Lea Ann Macknally and Philip Morris helped me describe elements of urban design. Beth Maynor Young's books and photography continue to inspire me to get out and experience our great natural assets.

I could list so many people and organizations who've been instrumental in protecting and expanding green space, such as Wendy Jackson and the Freshwater Land Trust, The Nature Conservancy, the Cahaba River Society, Black Warrior Riverkeeper, Forever Wild, the Community Foundation of Greater Birmingham, and Birmingham Urban Mountain Pedalers.

But most fundamental to this effort has been the support of my family. My parents, Clifford and Rita Spencer, always encouraged me to get outside and made possible so many adventures, particularly through participation in the Boy Scouts of America.

My wife, Ivy, has been incredibly patient and supportive in this journey, and my children, Peter, James, and Anna, have made my quest much richer, as they shared many of these hikes with me. Anna, in particular, served as my chief assistant photographer. I hope you'll find the same measure of reward that we did.

—*Thomas Spencer*

Preface

AS I WRITE, new trails are being blazed in Birmingham.

They're being cut through privet and kudzu on old iron ore–mining sites at Red Mountain Park. They're snaking along the Cahaba River and reclaiming the banks of other long-neglected urban streams.

In the heart of the city, earth movers are mounding dirt into new contours, turning an abandoned rail corridor into a crosstown trail for walkers, runners, and bicyclists.

As part of that project, in a cooperative venture between the city and the Rotary Club of Birmingham, a replica of the MAGIC CITY sign that once greeted passengers arriving at Birmingham's Terminal Station will be erected at the path's 20th Street trailhead.

That makes a statement, I think, about what we are now about as a city: that we value green space, the outdoors, and active living, and that we're working cooperatively to make better use of and take better care of our shared spaces—urban, suburban, and wilderness.

Birmingham in the 19th and 20th centuries was built on natural resources: iron ore, coal, and limestone. These assets, the principal ingredients for making iron and steel, were mined from the mountains and valleys and moved to mills and furnaces on a web of railroads.

The more you walk in the footprints of these endeavors, the more you're awed by the scale of them; by the ingenious engineering it took to design and build them; and by the sweat and strength of the labor that moved mountains, dug endless miles of underground tunnels, and melted rock in metal.

As we've moved into the 21st century and beyond our smoky industrial past, we're finding a different kind of value in our natural blessings. We're returning to our mountains and rivers to witness nature's resilience and endurance. And we draw on some of that spirit to revive ourselves. We're finding that in addition to our mineral

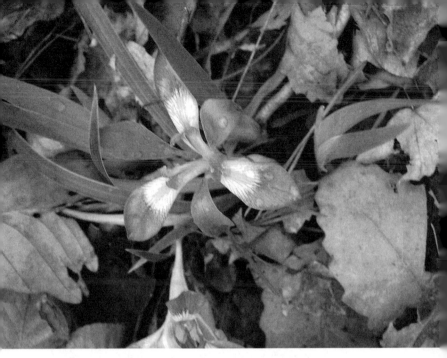

WILD IRIS BLOOMS IN SPRING AT MOSS ROCK PRESERVE. *(See Hikes 9–11.)*

wealth, this spot on the map has been blessed with a wealth of biodiversity, a variety of life found in few other places. We're doing more to protect it and celebrate it.

We're also blazing trails through our city's civil rights history and along the route finding inspiration in the courage that made us a better city and a better country.

As we've added new outdoor venues and expanded existing ones, it's been amazing to watch the trails fill with people hungry for fresh air and a fresh look at our native landscape.

Consider all we've done since the turn of the century: paved Vulcan Trail; restored Vulcan Park; and established Aldridge Gardens, Cahaba River National Wildlife Refuge, Moss Rock Preserve, Railroad Park, Red Mountain Park, and Turkey Creek Nature Preserve.

Trails at Ruffner Mountain Nature Preserve, Tannehill Ironworks Historical State Park, and Oak Mountain State Park have been significantly expanded and improved. The Shades Creek Greenway was constructed in Homewood, with links established to greenways along the creek in Mountain Brook. Other greenways are being built or planned along the Cahaba River in Trussville and Irondale, and along Five Mile Creek, Village Creek, and Valley Creek.

Farther afield, there are new facilities and better access to natural wonders at Little River Canyon National Preserve, the Sipsey Wilderness, Cheaha State Park, and Barton's Beach and Perry Lakes Park on the Cahaba.

In Anniston, a former railroad line is now the Chief Ladiga Trail, on which you can ride almost 100 miles from Anniston to the outskirts of Atlanta. Anniston's Coldwater Mountain now boasts a world-class mountain biking course on its peaks.

Perhaps most audacious of all, the Pinhoti Trail, the long-distance hiking trail that traverses the ridges of the Talladega National Forest, is now connected through Georgia to the southern terminus of the Appalachian Trail at Springer Mountain. A hiker can start at the southernmost Appalachian mountain—Flagg Mountain, near Sylacauga—and trek to Maine.

It's a great time to take a walk.

Don't wait until your kids get older; they can handle more than you think. Don't listen to their complaints about hiking; they'll forget them 5 minutes into the woods.

Don't wait for perfect weather. Rain, or just after, is the ideal time to see waterfalls. When it's cold, you can go for miles without breaking a sweat. When it's hot, we've got plenty of hikes that can end in a plunge into cool water. In the spring, you'll catch the early wildflowers. In the summer, the cicadas sing all day. In the fall, you get the colors, and in the winter, the great views.

There are weekends in the fall when you can trust that the Tide or Tigers will win even if you aren't watching. Surely once a season, you can clear your calendar of practices and games. I guarantee the family will better remember a trip to the Sipsey Wilderness than a run-of-the-mill weekend at the sports fields.

We tend to think we have to take an out-of-state vacation to see natural wonders.

Instead, drive an hour south to the Cahaba River National Wildlife Refuge. If you've ever spent a dawn at the tumbling shoals when the Cahaba lilies are in bloom and a blue heron is wading through the mist rising from the river, you've glimpsed Eden.

Trek along longleaf-pine ridges in the Talladega National Forest, among the grasses and wildflowers that have sprung back from the char of a prescribed burn.

Take in a sunset at Ruffner Mountain's Hawk's View. Ascend to the throne at King's Chair at Oak Mountain, or stand out on the rocky ledge at McDill Point at Cheaha. You'll feel high and grand.

At the base of Little River Canyon, you'll be awed by what a river's patient power can do over the course of millennia. And you'll realize you're a passenger in this tiny drop of time.

You probably won't see a vermilion darter when you visit Turkey Creek Nature Preserve, but you'll feel proud that we're trying to protect the habitat of this tiny endangered fish that God decorated with every color of the rainbow.

If you see mussels and snails in the Cahaba River, you likely won't be able to identify the species, but you'll know there's more variety in our rivers than nearly anywhere else on the planet.

You may see a bald eagle at Perry Lakes Park on the Cahaba, but if you go to the Wheeler National Wildlife Refuge at the right time of year, I guarantee you'll see a throng of lovely and charismatic sandhill cranes. With a little luck and planning, you could very well see whooping cranes, one of the world's most magnificent and most endangered species of bird.

It's a great time to take a walk.

And it's a great time to contribute your money or your labor. New trails don't just happen. Especially here in Alabama, anything that gets done involves individual donors, foundations, nonprofits, and hardworking volunteers.

Virtually every venue has a group of friends who help create, maintain, or improve the parks. If you hike in Alabama, it's hard to miss the contribution the Boy Scouts have made. Statewide trail

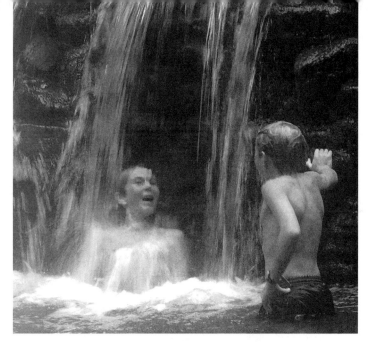

COOLING OFF IN A WATERFALL AT HURRICANE CREEK PARK *(see Hike 31)*

groups work all over to clear your way through the woods. Conservation groups work tirelessly to protect special places and the wider environment that sustains us and inspires us.

In compiling this book, I've pitched in and ventured out. I found that whatever energy I expended in those pursuits was returned to me many times over.

William Bartram, the great American naturalist of the 18th century, explored the country, including Alabama, cataloging species then new to science. He wrote that he was "continually impelled by a restless spirit of curiosity in pursuit of new productions of nature," adding that "my chief happiness consists in tracing and admiring the infinite power, majesty, and perfection of the great almighty Creator. . . ."

Catch that spirit. You'll get up in the morning wondering whether those flowers you saw yesterday bloomed overnight. You'll ask yourself how much water is tumbling down Peavine Falls today. Will this be the day the autumn leaves reach their peak of glory? And you'll want to go see. These are things you can't record and watch later. You've got to go.

Hiking
Recommendations

Best for Dogs
Red Mountain Park, Ruffner Mountain Nature Preserve

Best for Fall Color
Anything in and around Cheaha State Park, King's Chair at Oak Mountain State Park, Little River Canyon, Palisades Park, Ridge & Valley Loop at Ruffner Mountain

Best for Geology
Moss Rock Preserve, Red Mountain Park, Ruffner Mountain, Tannehill Ironworks Historical State Park

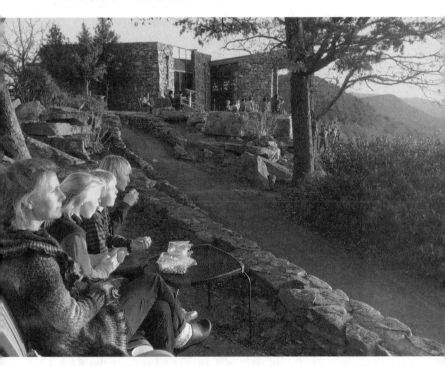

TAKING IN THE SUNSET AND FALL FOLIAGE AT CHEAHA STATE PARK *(see Hike 26)*

Best for History

Birmingham Civil Rights Heritage Trail, Irondale Furnace, Oak Hill Cemetery, Railroad Park, Red Mountain Park, Tannehill Ironworks Historical State Park

Best for Kids

Barton's Beach, Cahaba River National Wildlife Refuge, Railroad Park

Best for Scenery

The Blue Trail at Oak Mountain, Cheaha State Park and vicinity, Little River Canyon, Tree House to Hawk's View at Ruffner Mountain, the Sipsey Wilderness

Best for Seclusion

The Pinhoti Trail in the Talladega National Forest

Best for Waterfalls

The Chinnabee Silent Trail, Hurricane Creek Park, Little River Canyon, Moss Rock Preserve, Peavine Falls, Turkey Creek Falls

Best for Wildflowers

Aldridge Gardens, Homewood Forest Preserve, Moss Rock Waterfall Loop, Ruffner Mountain

Best for Wildlife

Barton's Beach and Perry Lakes Park in summer, Wheeler National Wildlife Refuge in January

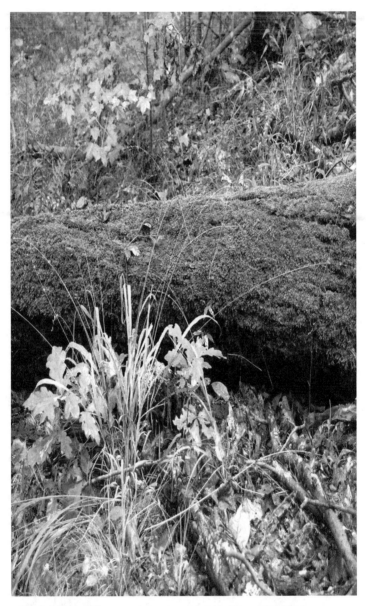

A MOSSY LOG ALONG THE BLUE TRAIL AT OAK MOUNTAIN STATE PARK
(see Hikes 12–15)

Introduction

About This Book

THE HIKES IN THIS BOOK are grouped both by geography and according to major hiking destinations. The **City Center** section contains hikes in and around downtown Birmingham; the **Suburbs** section includes hikes in communities just over Red Mountain from the city. **Ruffner Mountain Nature Preserve, Red Mountain Park, Moss Rock Preserve,** and **Oak Mountain State Park** merited sections of their own. Hikes south of the city, down I-59/I-20, take you to the river country, where the mountains fall away to the **Cahaba River.** The eastern attractions are generally reachable via I-20 (with the exception of **Flagg Mountain,** which is southeast down US 280) and take you into the sharper-edged **Talladega Mountain.** Hikes northwest of the city, reachable by going north on I-65, take you into the shady shelter coves of the **Sipsey Wilderness** as well as to other stops in that direction. The northeastern attractions, up AL 75, AL 79, or I-59, take you as far as **Little River Canyon** but also include stops closer to town in the rising plateaus of the Appalachians.

I chose these hikes because they are easily accessible and offer a good introduction to the diverse landscape and rich history that surround Birmingham. Each has its own particular qualities. Few, if any, would be rated at five stars in all five categories (see "Star Ratings," page 4). Some have great scenery but would be a slog for kids; others might be extremely convenient and kid-friendly but possibly crowded.

How to Use This Guidebook

The following section walks you through this guidebook's organization, making it easy and convenient to plan great hikes.

Overview Map, Map Key & Map Legend

The overview map on the inside front cover shows the primary trailheads for all 35 hikes. The numbers on the overview map pair with the map key on the facing page. A legend explaining the map symbols used throughout the book appears on the inside back cover.

Trail Maps

In addition to the overview map on the inside cover, a detailed map of each hike's route appears with its profile. On each of these maps, symbols indicate the trailhead, the complete route, significant features, facilities, and topographic landmarks such as creeks, overlooks, and peaks.

To produce the highly accurate maps in this book, I used a handheld GPS unit to gather data while hiking each route, then sent that data to Menasha Ridge Press's expert cartographers. Be aware, though, that your GPS device is no substitute for sound, sensible navigation that takes into account the conditions that you observe while hiking.

Further, despite the high quality of the maps in this guidebook, the publisher and I strongly recommend that you always carry an additional map, such as the ones noted in each profile opener's "Maps" listing.

Elevation Profile

For trails with significant changes in elevation, the hike descriptions include this graphical element. Entries for fairly flat routes, such the walk around Railroad Park (see page 35), do *not* display an elevation profile. Also, each entry's key information lists the elevation at the start of that specific route to its highest point; some hikes list additional elevations at notable points of interest.

For hike descriptions that include an elevation profile, this diagram represents the rises and falls of the trail as viewed from the side, over the complete distance (in miles) of that trail. On the diagram's vertical axis, or height scale, the number of feet indicated between each tick mark lets you visualize the climb. So that flat hikes don't look steep and vice versa, varying height scales provide an accurate image of each hike's climbing challenge. For example, one hike might

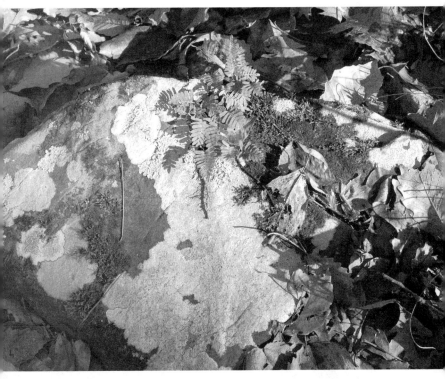

LICHENS, MOSS, AND FERNS FESTOON A BOULDER AT OAK MOUNTAIN IN WINTER.

rise to 2,407 feet at Mount Cheaha, while an even more challenging hike at Oak Mountain might top out at 1,200 feet above sea level.

The Hike Profile

Each profile opens with the hike's star ratings, GPS trailhead coordinates, and other key at-a-glance information—from the trail's distance and configuration to phone numbers and websites. (Some of this key info is provided in the area overviews preceding each section's hikes.) Each profile also includes a map (see "Trail Maps," previous page). The main text for each profile includes four sections: Overview, Route Details, Nearby Attractions (where applicable), and Directions (for getting to the trailhead area).

STAR RATINGS

Here's how they break down for the following five categories:

SCENERY:

★ ★ ★ ★ ★	Unique, picturesque panoramas
★ ★ ★ ★	Diverse vistas
★ ★ ★	Pleasant views
★ ★	Unchanging landscape
★	Not selected for scenery

TRAIL CONDITION:

★ ★ ★ ★ ★	Consistently well maintained
★ ★ ★ ★	Stable, with no surprises
★ ★ ★	Average terrain to negotiate
★ ★	Inconsistent, with good and poor areas
★	Rocky, overgrown, or often muddy

CHILDREN:

★ ★ ★ ★ ★	Babes in strollers are welcome
★ ★ ★ ★	Fun for any kid past the toddler stage
★ ★ ★	Good for young hikers with proven stamina
★ ★	Not enjoyable for children
★	Not advisable for children

DIFFICULTY:

★ ★ ★ ★ ★	Grueling
★ ★ ★ ★	Strenuous
★ ★ ★	Moderate: won't beat you up—but you'll know you've been hiking
★ ★	Easy, with patches of moderate
★	Good for a relaxing stroll

SOLITUDE:

★ ★ ★ ★ ★	Positively tranquil
★ ★ ★ ★	Spurts of isolation
★ ★ ★	Moderately secluded
★ ★	Crowded on weekends and holidays
★	Steady stream of individuals and/or groups

GPS TRAILHEAD COORDINATES

As noted in "Trail Maps" (page 2), I used a handheld GPS unit to obtain geographic data and sent the information to the cartographers at Menasha Ridge. In the opener for each hike profile, the coordinates—the intersection of latitude (north) and longitude (west)—will orient you from the trailhead. In some cases, you can drive within viewing distance of a trailhead. Other hiking routes require a short walk to the trailhead from a parking area.

This guidebook expresses GPS coordinates in degree–decimal minute format. The latitude–longitude grid system is likely quite familiar to you, but here's a refresher, pertinent to visualizing the coordinates:

Imaginary lines of latitude—called *parallels* and approximately 69 miles apart from each other—run horizontally around the globe. The equator is established to be 0°, and each parallel is indicated by degrees from the equator: up to 90°N at the North Pole, and down to 90°S at the South Pole.

Imaginary lines of longitude—called *meridians*—run perpendicular to lines of latitude and are likewise indicated by degrees. Starting from 0° at the Prime Meridian in Greenwich, England, they continue to the east and west until they meet 180° later at the International Date Line in the Pacific Ocean. At the equator, longitude lines also are approximately 69 miles apart, but that distance narrows as the meridians converge toward the North and South Poles.

To convert GPS coordinates given in degrees, minutes, and seconds to degrees and decimal minutes, divide the seconds by 60. For more on GPS technology, visit **usgs.gov.**

DISTANCE & CONFIGURATION

Distance indicates the length of the hike round-trip, from start to finish. If the hike description includes options to shorten or extend the hike, those round-trip distances are also factored here. *Configuration* defines the type of route—for example, an out-and-back (which takes you in and out the same way), a point-to-point (or one-way route), a figure-eight, or a balloon.

HIKING TIME

A speed of 2–3 miles per hour is a general rule of thumb for hiking the trails in this book, depending on the terrain and whether you have children with you. That pace typically allows time for taking photos, for dawdling and admiring views, and for alternating stretches of hills and descents. When deciding whether or not to follow a particular trail in this guidebook, consider your own pace, the weather, your general physical condition, and your energy level on a given day.

HIGHLIGHTS

Lists features that draw hikers to the trail: waterfalls, historic sites, and the like.

ELEVATION

In each hike's key information, you will see the elevation (in feet) at the trailhead and another figure for the high (or low) point on the trail; where appropriate, additional elevations are also listed. For routes that involve significant ascents and descents, the hike profile also includes an elevation diagram (see page 2).

ACCESS

Fees or permits required to hike the trail are detailed here—and noted if there are none. Trail-access hours are also listed here.

MAPS

Resources for maps, in addition to those in this guidebook, are listed here. As noted earlier, we recommend that you carry more than one map—and that you consult those maps before heading out on the trail in order to resolve any confusion or discrepancy.

FACILITIES

Includes restrooms, phones, water, picnic tables, and other basics at or near the trailhead.

WHEELCHAIR ACCESS

Notes paved sections or other areas where one can safely use a wheelchair.

COMMENTS

Here you'll find assorted nuggets of information, such as whether or not dogs are allowed on the trails.

CONTACTS

Listed here are phone numbers and websites for checking trail conditions and gleaning other day-to-day information.

Overview, Route Details, Nearby Attractions & Directions

These four elements compose the heart of the hike. "Overview" gives you a quick summary of what to expect on that trail; "Route Details" guides you on the hike, from start to finish; "Nearby Attractions" suggests appealing adjacent sites, such as restaurants, museums, and other trails (note that not every hike profile has these). "Directions" will get you to the trailhead from a well-known road or highway; for some City Center hikes, the nearest cross streets are provided.

Weather

The following chart provides a month-by-month snapshot of the weather in the Birmingham area. For each month, "Hi Temp" shows the average daytime high, "Lo Temp" gives the average nighttime low, and "Rain or Snow" lists the average precipitation.

MONTH	HI TEMP	LO TEMP	RAIN or SNOW
January	54°F	34°F	4.84"
February	59°F	37°F	4.70"
March	67°F	44°F	5.23"
April	74°F	51°F	4.38"
May	82°F	60°F	4.99"
June	88°F	68°F	4.38"
July	91°F	72°F	4.80"
August	91°F	71°F	3.93"
September	85°F	64°F	3.90"
October	75°F	53°F	3.44"
November	65°F	44°F	4.85"
December	56°F	36°F	4.45"

Water

How much is enough? Well, one simple physiological fact should convince you to err on the side of excess when deciding how much water to pack: a hiker walking steadily in 90° heat needs about 10 quarts of fluid per day—that's 2.5 gallons. A good rule of thumb is to hydrate prior to your hike, carry (and drink) 6 ounces of water for every mile you plan to hike, and hydrate again after the hike. For most people, the pleasures of hiking make carrying water a relatively minor price to pay to remain safe and healthy, so pack more water than you anticipate needing, even for short hikes.

If you're tempted to drink "found water," do so with extreme caution. Many ponds and lakes you'll encounter are fairly stagnant, and the water tastes terrible. Drinking such water presents inherent risks for thirsty trekkers. Giardia parasites contaminate many water sources and cause the dreaded intestinal ailment giardiasis, which can last for weeks after onset. For more information, visit **cdc.gov /parasites/giardia.**

In any case, effective treatment is essential before you use any water source found along the trail. Boiling water for 2–3 minutes is always a safe measure for camping, but day hikers can consider iodine tablets, approved chemical mixes, filtration units rated for giardia, and ultraviolet filtration. Some of these methods (for example, filtration with an added carbon filter) remove bad tastes typical in stagnant water, while others add their own taste. As a precaution, carry a means of water purification in case you ever underestimate your consumption needs.

Clothing

Weather, unexpected trail conditions, fatigue, extended hiking duration, and wrong turns can individually or collectively turn a great outing into a very uncomfortable one at best—and a life-threatening one at worst. Thus, proper attire plays a key role in staying comfortable and, sometimes, in staying alive. Some helpful guidelines:

★ Choose silk, wool, or synthetics for maximum comfort in all of your hiking attire—from hats to socks and in between. Cotton is fine if the weather remains dry and stable, but you won't be happy if that material gets wet.

★ Always wear a hat, or at least tuck one into your day pack or hitch it to your belt. Hats offer all-weather sun and wind protection as well as warmth if it turns cold.

★ Be ready to layer up or down as the day progresses and the mercury rises or falls. Today's outdoor wear makes layering easy, with such designs as jackets that convert to vests and zip-off or button-up legs.

★ Mosquitoes, poison ivy, and thorny bushes found along many trails can generate short-term discomfort and long-term agony. When temperatures permit, a lightweight pair of pants and a long-sleeved shirt can go a long way toward protecting you from these pests.

★ Wear hiking boots or sturdy hiking sandals with toe protection. Flip-flopping along a paved urban greenway is one thing, but you should never hike a trail in open sandals or casual sneakers. Your bones and arches need support, and your skin needs protection.

★ Pair that footwear with good socks. If you prefer not to sheathe your feet when wearing hiking sandals, tuck the socks into your day pack—you may need them if temperatures plummet or if you hit rocky turf and pebbles begin to irritate your feet. And if it's cold and you've lost your gloves, you can adapt the socks into mittens.

★ Don't leave rainwear behind, even if the day dawns clear and sunny. Tuck into your day pack, or tie around your waist, a jacket that's breathable and either water-resistant or waterproof. Investigate different choices at your local outdoors retailer. If you're a frequent hiker, you'll ideally have more than one rainwear weight, material, and style in your closet to protect you in all seasons in your regional climate and hiking microclimates.

Essential Gear

Today you can buy outdoor vests that have up to 20 pockets shaped and sized to carry everything from toothpicks to binoculars. Or, if you don't aspire to feel like a burro, you can neatly stow all of these items in your day pack or backpack. The following list showcases never-hike-without-them items—in alphabetical order, as all are important:

★ *Extra food:* trail mix, granola bars, or other high-energy snacks.

★ *Extra clothes:* raingear, a change of socks, and depending on the season, a warm hat and gloves.

★ *Flashlight or headlamp* with extra bulb and batteries.

★ *Insect repellent.* For some areas and seasons, this is vital.

★ *Maps and a high-quality compass.* Even if you know the terrain from previous hikes, don't leave home without these tools. And, as previously noted, bring maps in addition to those in this guidebook, and consult your maps prior to the hike. If you're GPS-savvy, bring that device, too, but don't rely on it as your sole navigational tool—battery life is limited, after all—and be sure to check its accuracy against that of your maps and compass.

★ *Pocketknife and/or multitool.*

★ *Sunscreen.* Check the expiration date on the tube or bottle.

★ *Water.* As we've emphasized more than once, bring more than you think you'll drink. Depending on your destination, you may want to bring a container and iodine or a filter for purifying water in case you run out.

★ *Whistle.* It could become your best friend in an emergency.

★ *Windproof matches and/or a lighter,* as well as a fire starter.

First-Aid Kit

In addition to the preceding items, those that follow may seem daunting to carry along for a day hike. But any paramedic will tell you that the products listed here—again, in alphabetical order, because all are important—are just the basics. The reality of hiking is that you can be out for a week of backpacking and acquire only a mosquito bite. Or you can hike for an hour, slip, and suffer a cut or broken bone. Fortunately, the items listed pack into a very small space. You can also buy convenient prepackaged kits at your pharmacy or online.

★ Adhesive bandages

★ Antibiotic ointment (such as Neosporin)

★ Aspirin, acetaminophen (Tylenol), or ibuprofen (Advil)

★ Athletic tape

★ Blister kit (moleskin or an adhesive variety such as Spenco 2nd Skin)

★ Butterfly-closure bandages

★ Diphenhydramine (Benadryl), in case of allergic reactions

★ Elastic bandages (such as Ace) or joint wraps (such as Spenco)

★ Epinephrine in a prefilled syringe (EpiPen), typically by prescription only, for people known to have severe allergic reactions to hiking mishaps such as bee stings

★ Gauze (one roll and a half-dozen 4-by-4-inch pads)

★ Hydrogen peroxide or iodine

Note: Consider your intended terrain and the number of hikers in your party before you exclude any article listed above. A short stroll may not inspire you to carry a complete kit, but anything beyond that warrants precaution. When hiking alone, you should always be prepared for a medical need. And if you're a twosome or with a group, one or more people in your party should be equipped with first-aid material.

General Safety

The following tips may have the familiar ring of Mom's voice:

★ *Always let someone know where you'll be hiking and how long you expect to be gone.* It's a good idea to give that person a copy of your route, particularly if you're headed into any isolated area. Let him or her know when you return.

★ *Always sign in and out of any trail registers provided.* Don't hesitate to comment on the trail condition if space is provided; that's your opportunity to alert others to any problems you encounter.

★ *Don't count on a cell phone for your safety.* Reception may be spotty or nonexistent on the trail, even on an urban walk—especially one embraced by towering trees.

★ *Always carry food and water, even for a short hike.* And bring more water than you think you'll need. (We can't emphasize this enough.)

★ *Ask questions.* Public-land employees are on hand to help. It's a lot easier to solicit advice before a problem occurs, and it will help you avoid a mishap away from civilization when it's too late to amend an error.

★ *Stay on designated trails.* Even on the most clearly marked trails, you usually reach a point where you have to stop and consider in which direction to head. If you become disoriented, don't panic. As soon as you think you may be off-track, stop, assess your current direction, and then retrace your steps to the point where you went astray. Using a map, a compass, and this book, and keeping in mind what you've passed thus far, reorient yourself, and trust your judgment on which way to continue. If you become absolutely unsure of how to continue, return to your vehicle the way you came in. Should you become completely lost and have no idea how to find the trailhead, remaining in place along the trail and waiting for help is most often the best option for adults, and always the best option for children.

★ *Always carry a whistle,* another precaution that we can't overemphasize. It may become a lifesaver if you get lost or hurt.

★ *Be especially careful when crossing streams.* Whether you're fording the stream or crossing on a log, make every step count. If you have any doubt about maintaining your balance on a log, ford the stream instead: use a trekking pole or stout stick for balance and *face upstream as you cross.* If a stream seems too deep to ford, turn back. Whatever is on the other side isn't worth risking your life for.

★ *Be careful at overlooks.* While these areas may provide spectacular views, they are potentially hazardous. Stay back from the edge of outcrops, and make absolutely sure of your footing—a misstep can mean a nasty and possibly fatal fall.

★ *Standing dead trees and storm-damaged living trees pose a significant hazard to hikers.* These trees may have loose or broken limbs that could fall at any time. While walking beneath trees, and when choosing a spot to rest or enjoy your snack, *look up.*

★ *Know the symptoms of subnormal body temperature, or hypothermia.* Shivering and forgetfulness are the two most common indicators of this stealthy killer. Hypothermia can occur at any elevation, even in the summer, especially when the hiker is wearing lightweight cotton clothing. If symptoms develop, get to shelter, hot liquids, and dry clothes ASAP.

★ *Likewise, know the symptoms of heat exhaustion, or hyperthermia.* Lightheadedness and loss of energy are the first two indicators. If you feel these symptoms, find some shade, drink your water, remove as many layers of clothing as practical, and stay put until you cool down. Marching through heat exhaustion leads to heatstroke—which can be deadly. If you should be sweating and you're not, that's the signature warning sign. Your hike is over at that point: heatstroke is a life-threatening condition that can cause seizures, convulsions, and eventually death. If you or a companion reaches that point, do whatever you can to cool down, and seek medical attention immediately.

★ *Most importantly, take along your brain.* A cool, calculating mind is the single most important asset on the trail. Think before you act. Watch your step. Plan ahead. Avoiding accidents before they happen is the best way to ensure a rewarding and relaxing hike.

Watchwords for Flora & Fauna

Hikers should remain aware of the following concerns regarding plant life and wildlife, described in alphabetical order.

MOSQUITOES Ward off these pests with insect repellent and/or repellent-impregnated clothing. In some areas, mosquitoes are known to carry the West Nile virus, so all due caution should be taken to avoid their bites.

POISON IVY, OAK & SUMAC Recognizing and avoiding these plants are the most effective ways to prevent the painful, itchy rashes associated with them. Poison ivy occurs as a vine or groundcover, three leaflets to a leaf; poison oak occurs as either a vine or shrub, also with three leaflets; and poison sumac flourishes in swampland, each leaf having 7–13 leaflets. Urushiol, the oil in the sap of these plants, is responsible for the rash. Within 14 hours of exposure,

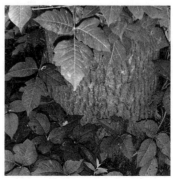

Photo: Tom Watson

raised lines and/or blisters will appear on your skin, accompanied by a terrible itch. Try to refrain from scratching, though, because bacteria under your fingernails can cause an infection. Wash and dry the affected area thoroughly, applying calamine lotion to help dry out the rash. If the itching or blistering is severe, seek medical attention. To keep from spreading the misery to someone else, wash not only any exposed parts of your body but also any oil-contaminated clothes, hiking gear, and pets.

SNAKES Rattlesnakes, cottonmouths, copperheads, and corals are among the most common venomous snakes in the United States, and their hibernation season is typically October–April. But despite their fearsome reputation, rattlesnakes like to bask in the sun and won't bite unless threatened.

In the Birmingham area, you could encounter any of the snakes listed above, though coral snakes are exceedingly rare. The snakes you'll most likely see are nonvenomous species and subspecies. The best rule is to leave all snakes alone, give them a wide berth as you hike past, and make sure your hiking companions (including dogs) do the same.

When hiking, stick to well-used trails, and wear over-the-ankle boots and loose-fitting long pants. Don't step or put your hands beyond your range of detailed visibility, and avoid wandering around in the dark. Step *onto* logs and rocks, never *over* them, and be especially careful when climbing rocks. Always avoid walking through dense brush or willow thickets, and be alert crossing creeks—cottonmouths spend much of their time in the water and are territorial.

TICKS These arachnids are often found on brush and tall grass, where they seem to be waiting to hitch a ride on warm-blooded passersby. Adult ticks are most active April–May and again October–November. The black-legged (deer) tick is the primary carrier of Lyme disease.

A few precautions: Wear light-colored clothing, which will make it easy for you to spot ticks before they migrate to your skin. When your hike is done, visually check your hair, the back of your neck, your armpits, and your socks. During your posthike shower, take a moment to do a more complete body check. Use tweezers to remove a tick that is already embedded. Treat the bite with disinfectant solution.

Hunting

A number of rules, regulations, and licenses govern Alabama's various hunting types and their related seasons. Though no problems generally arise, hikers may wish to forgo their trips during big-game seasons, when the woods suddenly seem filled with orange and camouflage. Deer-hunting season generally runs from November through January. Turkey hunting takes place in November (in some areas also December and January) and in March and April. Hunters may be pursuing various small-game species from September through the end of February. For more information, visit **outdooralabama.com/hunting.**

Trail Etiquette

Always treat trails, wildlife, and fellow hikers with respect. Here are some reminders:

★ Plan ahead in order to be self-sufficient at all times. For example, carry necessary supplies for changes in weather or other conditions. A well-planned trip brings satisfaction to you and to others.

★ Hike on open trails only.

★ In seasons or construction areas where road or trail closures may be a possibility, use the websites or phone numbers listed in the "Contacts" section at the beginning of each hike profile to check conditions before you head out for your hike. And don't try to circumvent such closures.

★ Avoid trespassing on private land, and obtain all permits and authorization as required. Also, leave gates as you found them or as directed by signage.

★ Be courteous to other hikers, bikers, equestrians, and others you encounter on the trails.

★ Never spook wild animals or pets. An unannounced approach, a sudden movement, or a loud noise startles most critters, and a surprised animal can be dangerous to you, to others, and to itself. Give animals plenty of space.

★ Observe the YIELD signs around the region's trailheads and back-country. Typically they advise hikers to yield to horses, and bikers to yield to both horses and hikers. Observing common courtesy on hills, hikers and bikers yield to any uphill traffic. When encountering mounted riders or horsepackers, hikers can courteously step off the trail, on the downhill side if possible. So that horses can see and hear you, calmly greet their riders before they reach you, and do not dart behind trees. Also resist the urge to pet horses unless you are invited to do so.

★ Stay on the existing trail, and do not blaze any new trails.

★ Pack out what you pack in, leaving only your footprints. No one likes to see the trash someone else has left behind. Bring a trash bag with you, and pick up after others when possible.

Tips for Enjoying Hiking in Birmingham

Yes, Birmingham and the surrounding areas can get hot and humid in the summer, but many of these hikes feature waterways to cool off in. Besides, it's healthy to sweat. Our winters are mild; days after a hard freeze, you'll generally find temperatures in the 50s and 60s. Get out in it, especially since wintertime usually features the best flow in local waterfalls. Fall is glorious, and in the spring wildflowers emerge quickly before the thick canopy closes in. So get out early and often.

A WATERFALL TUCKED AWAY IN BOULDER CANYON, NEAR THE VESTAVIA HILLS LIBRARY IN THE FOREST *(see Hike 8)*

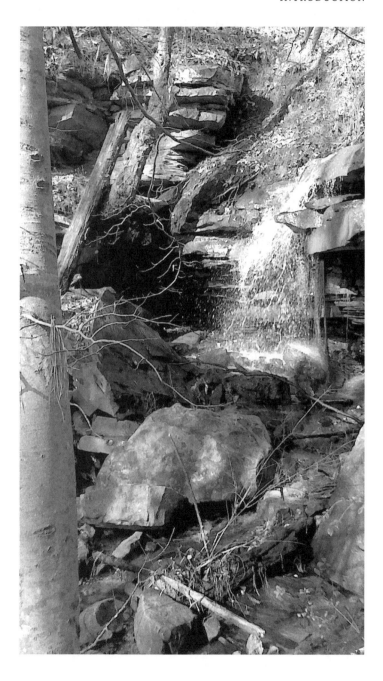

City Center (Hikes 1–4)

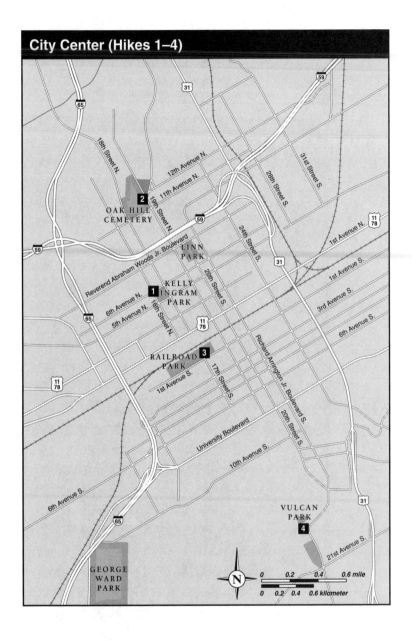

City Center

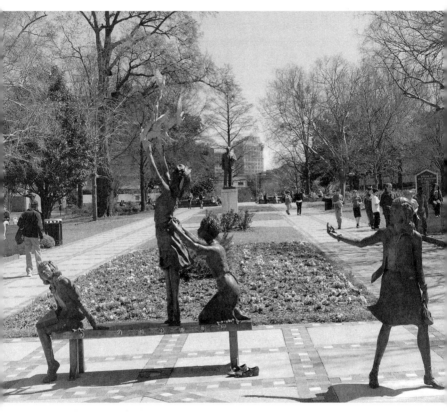

THESE STATUES IN KELLY INGRAM PARK COMMEMORATE THE FOUR GIRLS
KILLED IN THE BOMBING OF SIXTEENTH STREET BAPTIST CHURCH IN 1963.
(See Hike 1.)

City Center Overview

FOR A LONG TIME, Birmingham's city center was a place you drove into and out of. There wasn't much living downtown, and there wasn't much walking downtown.

That has changed. Early mornings and late afternoons, you see urbanites, not dressed in business attire, strolling or striding, pushing strollers and walking dogs.

At 6 p.m. on various evenings through the spring and summer, daytime bankers, nurses, architects, and lawyers wander down to **Railroad Park** for community Crunk, Bootcamp, Zumba, and yoga classes. When the Birmingham Barons are in town, people converge from every direction on the new **Regions Field.**

Crews are at work right now on a crosstown trail—a collaboration between the city of Birmingham and the Rotary Club of Birmingham—that will begin to better link Railroad Park to Sloss Furnaces, the Lakeview District, and, later, Avondale.

On the Southside over the past decade, the **University of Alabama at Birmingham** has been transformed from a commuter college clogged with cars into an urban university, with academic buildings and residence halls clustered around a large, grassy quadrangle, UAB Green. The city, UAB, and Children's Hospital have plans to further improve pedestrian and bicycle connections from the university and the medical district to Railroad Park.

You can find a visionary version of what Birmingham could look like for walkers, runners, and bicyclists at the website of the **Red Rock Ridge & Valley Trail System (redrocktrail.org)**. This is a master plan for an entire regional network of trails spreading out from downtown to the neighborhoods and beyond.

Trailheads and Trails

On the following pages are four hikes to get you started on your exploration of the city center. The first starts at ground zero for Birmingham's 1963 civil rights confrontation and follows trails that form an outdoor museum complementing the powerful displays inside the

20

Birmingham Civil Rights Institute. The second takes you through the city of Birmingham's original cemetery—the final resting place of city fathers such as J. W. Sloss, founder of Sloss Furnaces, and the Rev. Fred Shuttlesworth, the fearless preacher who led the charge against segregation. The third is a circuit around Railroad Park, Birmingham's new civic living room. The final hike is a loop from our iconic landmark, Vulcan, along the Vulcan Trail, down to the UAB campus, over to Five Points South, and back up the mountain.

Other City Center Attractions

ALABAMA THEATRE A classic movie palace, built in 1927 and lovingly restored to its former glory. Consult the website for concerts and classic movies. 1817 Third Ave. N.; 205-252-2262, **alabamatheatre.com.**

BIRMINGHAM MUSEUM OF ART Has one of the finest permanent collections in the Southeast. 2000 Rev. Abraham Woods Jr. Blvd.; 205-254-2565, **artsbma.org.**

BIRMINGHAM PUBLIC LIBRARY'S LINN-HENLEY RESEARCH LIBRARY On Linn Park, next to the Jefferson County Courthouse, it's worth a visit just to see the beautiful interior murals of mythological and fairy-tale characters. Research Southern or family history while you're here. 2100 Park Pl.; 205-226-3600, **bplonline.org.**

LYRIC FINE ARTS THEATRE A vaudeville theatre built in 1914, the Lyric is in the midst of a complete restoration. 1817 Third Ave. N.; 205-252-2262, **lightupthelyric.com.**

McWANE SCIENCE CENTER Interactive exhibits; Alabama dinosaurs, wildlife, and aquatic life; and IMAX movies just scratch the surface of what's available at the city's science headquarters. 200 19th St. N.; 205-714-8300, **mcwane.org.**

PEANUT DEPOT Visit this landmark that's been selling fresh-roasted peanuts for more than 100 years. 2016 Morris Ave.; 205-251-3314, **peanutdepot.com.**

SLOSS FURNACES NATIONAL HISTORIC LANDMARK Blast furnaces that were once a center of Birmingham's iron-making industry. Open for self-guided tours every day but Monday. 20 32nd St. N.; 205-324-1911, **slossfurnaces.com.**

Contacts and More Information

The nonprofit **City Action Patrol (CAP),** supported by downtown businesses, provides escorts and guides to downtown. They sport red shirts and black pants and ride bikes or patrol in vehicles, lending a layer of security and friendliness to the downtown experience. If you need directions or have a dead battery or flat tire, call CAP at 205-251-0111.

The **Greater Birmingham Convention & Visitors Bureau** offers a wealth of information on events and attractions downtown and beyond. A smartphone app, maps, and more are available at its website, **birminghamal.org.**

Comments

Downtown Birmingham is a city, not a gated community. It's beautifully landscaped and generally safe and well kept, but it's not immune to the realities of urban life. Be alert. Lock your car. It's probably best to stay out of the darker, more remote corners after dark. You may encounter homeless individuals, and they may ask for money. Give if you feel inclined, or politely decline and maybe later donate to one of the many ministries that help them find food and housing.

Civil Rights Heritage Trail:
Birmingham's Walk to Freedom

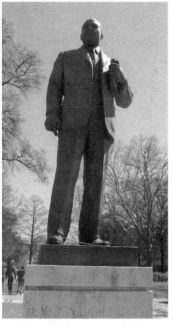

SCENERY: ★ ★ ★ ★ ★
TRAIL CONDITION: ★ ★ ★ ★
CHILDREN: ★ ★ ★
DIFFICULTY: ★
SOLITUDE: ★ ★

GPS TRAILHEAD COORDINATES:
N33° 30.983' W86° 48.862'

DISTANCE & CONFIGURATION: 1-mile out-and-back. Additional walking routes branch off this route.

HIKING TIME: You could power-walk the whole thing in less than an hour, but if you slow down and delve into the story, you could spend hours.

HIGHLIGHTS: Walk in the footsteps of men, women, and children who changed the world. See historic sites from the climactic battles of the civil rights movement, such as Sixteenth Street Baptist Church and Kelly Ingram Park. Appreciate the factual information, photos, and inspirational quotes on the signage that guides you through downtown and through history.

ELEVATION: Different routes vary between 591' and 606'.

ACCESS: Kelly Ingram Park and the self-guided street tours are accessible every day during daylight hours. The Birmingham Civil Rights Institute is open Tuesday–Saturday, 10 a.m.–5 p.m., and Sunday, 1–5 p.m.; open Monday from January 15 (Martin Luther King Jr.'s birthday) through the end of February; closed on major holidays. Admission is $12 for adults, with discounts for children, seniors, and others; no admission charge on Sunday, but donations are appreciated. Individual or group tours of Sixteenth Street Baptist Church are also available. To make reservations, call 205-251-9402; open by appointment only Tuesday–Friday, 10 a.m.–3 p.m., and Saturday, 10 a.m.–1 p.m.; admission is $5.

MAPS: Maps of the self-guided walking routes are still under development, though a version can be found online at **heritagetrail.birminghamal.gov.**

FACILITIES: The Birmingham Civil Rights Institute has restrooms. Kelly Ingram Park and Linn Park have benches, tables, and green space for picnicking.

WHEELCHAIR ACCESS: Yes

COMMENTS: Kelly Ingram Park, Linn Park, and the more remote areas of downtown are best toured during daylight hours.

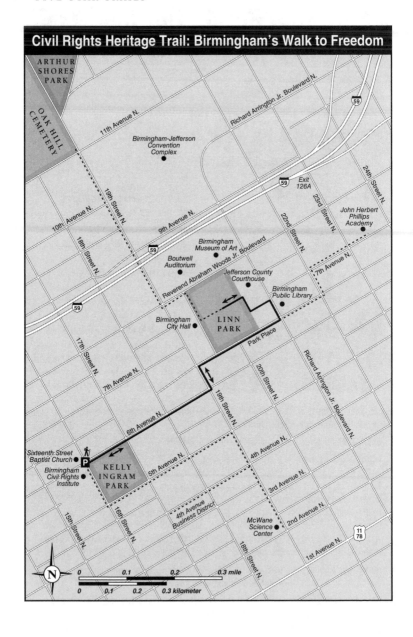

Civil Rights Heritage Trail: Birmingham's Walk to Freedom

CONTACTS: Birmingham Civil Rights Institute, 205-328-9696, **bcri.org.** Information on the self-guided street tours is available at **heritagetrail.birminghamal.gov.** Sixteenth Street Baptist Church, 205-251-9402, **16thstreetbaptist.org.**

Overview

During the run-up to and observation of the 50th anniversary of 1963's civil rights confrontations, the city of Birmingham launched the Civil Rights Heritage Trail, an effort to take history to the streets of downtown. There are now multiple self-guided routes through downtown, some featuring audio narration via cell phone. Kelly Ingram Park, the scene of the most famous clashes between protestors and law enforcement, serves as the trailhead for principal tour routes. Adjacent to the park are the Birmingham Civil Rights Institute, which commemorates the struggle against segregation, and the Sixteenth Street Baptist Church, a staging post for the marches and the target of a bombing on September 16, 1963, which killed four young black girls.

Route Details

Boston has its Freedom Trail, where in a short distance you can visit several of the most significant sites of the American Revolution. Jamestown and Williamsburg, Virginia, and Washington, DC, are also spots where you can walk through some of the most significant events in American history. But Birmingham has its own concentration of significant events in US history: the churches, homes, parks, and streets that saw some of the most famous events of the civil rights struggle.

Famous leaders such as Martin Luther King Jr. spoke from the pulpit of the Sixteenth Street Baptist Church and marched here. But also remembered are common people, both adults and children, who faced down police dogs and fire hoses and paved the way for the ultimate victory over legal segregation.

Start at the corner of 16th Street North and Sixth Avenue North. On one corner stands the **Birmingham Civil Rights Institute.** Standing near the entrance is a statue of Fred Shuttlesworth, the fearless leader of the

Birmingham movement and an influential figure in the wider struggle. A tour of the BCRI's comprehensive history exhibits can easily take up a well-spent afternoon. It will leave you with a mix of emotional exhaustion and uplift.

Across Sixth Avenue to the north is **Sixteenth Street Baptist Church,** where, in the spring of 1963, marchers rallied before heading out to face the forces of Eugene "Bull" Connor, Birmingham's notorious Commissioner of Public Safety. Later, on the morning of Sunday, September 15, 1963, the church was bombed by members of the Ku Klux Klan. Killed in the blast were Denise McNair, 11, Addie Mae Collins, 14, Carole Robertson, 14, and Cynthia Wesley, 14, who were in the church's basement dressing room, preparing for the 11 a.m. service. The act of terror shocked the conscience of the nation. The events in Birmingham in 1963 precipitated the passage of the landmark Civil Rights Act of 1964.

A statue of the four girls was installed and dedicated across the street at the entrance to **Kelly Ingram Park** in 2013. It's a good place to start your tour of the park, with its sculptures and water features. In the 1960s, Birmingham was divided. This area west of downtown was a center of black-owned businesses. Just blocks away to the east lay centers of white-dominated government and white-owned business and retail.

Urged on by Shuttlesworth, the leaders of the Southern Christian Leadership Conference decided to come to Birmingham to confront one of segregation's most tenacious defenders, the Bull Connor–led city government.

As the protests swelled and jails filled, Connor formed a perimeter east of the park in an effort to keep protests from reaching City Hall or the retail district. Attempting to corral and disperse the protestors, Connor deployed fire hoses and the police force's canine corps. The images of the snarling dogs and protesters being blasted with water cannons made newspapers and television broadcasts around the country and the world.

Statues in the park memorialize the confrontation, inviting visitors to imagine the courage it took to persist against such aggression. There is a large statue of King, and the flowing water in the fountains recalls his allusion, in his "I Have a Dream" speech, to the words of the prophet Amos: "We will not be satisfied," King said, "until justice rolls down like waters and righteousness like a mighty stream." Look for numbered signs around the park that describe how to access the audio tour by cell phone.

As a side note, the park is named for Osmond Kelly Ingram, an Oneonta native who was the first American sailor killed in action in World War I, aboard the USS *Cassin* on October 1, 1917. The park also has a monument to Birmingham native Julius Ellsberry, the first black Alabama man to die in World War II; he was killed at Pearl Harbor aboard the USS *Oklahoma* on December 7, 1941.

From the park, you have a choice of two downtown routes for self-guided tours: the **March to Government (Route A),** which follows the route marchers would have taken toward City Hall, or the **March to Retail (Route B),** which takes you to the scene of protests in what was once the center of retail shopping in Birmingham. Along the way, you'll pass the former Trailways bus terminal, where the Freedom Riders were beaten by a mob in 1961. On a lighter note, you'll return on Fourth Avenue North, where you'll find a statue of the singing group The Temptations, including Birmingham native Eddie Kendrick. This is part of the **Fourth Avenue Business District,** historically home to a concentration of businesses catering to the black community.

Because both routes are marked by highly visible signage that tells pieces of the civil rights story along the way, I won't provide turn-by-turn narration. Each route is about a mile, out-and-back. As a general tip, you can walk it one way digesting the information on the front of signs and looking for cues to tap into the audio tour. Coming back, you can read the larger quotes on the back sides of the signs, without having to pause as much. Each sign is numbered and has a small locator map on it, though generally you can spot your next stop by looking around.

The March to Government leaves Kelly Ingram Park and travels Sixth Avenue North to the east, turns left (north) on 19th Street North, and then right on Park Place headed toward Linn Park, the Jefferson County Courthouse, and Birmingham City Hall. Note a couple of things along the way not officially on the tour: One is the obelisk in Linn Park devoted to Confederate soldiers and sailors. The other is a statue of Thomas Jefferson alongside the county courthouse. Both serve as reminders that the struggle of 1963 was part of an enduring struggle for freedom.

From Linn Park, if you'd like take a longer walk, you can pick up the **March for Education (Route D).** It begins in the southeast corner of the park by the Birmingham Public Library and travels to **John Herbert Phillips Academy.** In 1957, Fred Shuttlesworth led a group of students in an attempt to enroll them and integrate Phillips, then an all-white high school. Shuttlesworth was brutally beaten by a mob in the attempt. Today, Phillips Academy is a pre-K- through eighth-grade school in the Birmingham city system.

Departing from the northwest corner of Linn Park is the **March to a Purposeful Life (Route E).** This route narrates Shuttlesworth's biography. It ends on 19th Street North, north of the Birmingham-Jefferson Convention Complex. Shuttlesworth is buried in **Oak Hill Cemetery** (see next hike), across the street from the trail's terminus.

Directions

The Birmingham Civil Rights Institute, Sixteenth Street Baptist Church, and Kelly Ingram Park are at the intersection of Sixth Avenue North and 16th Street North. Note that Birmingham streets are laid out in a grid: Streets run north–south, and avenues run east–west. The central rail corridor in downtown Birmingham marks the division between north and south. On the north side of the tracks, avenues increase numerically as you go north; streets decrease numerically as you travel from west to east.

Oak Hill Cemetery

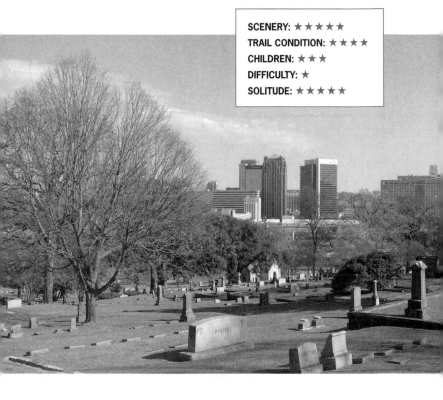

> SCENERY: ★ ★ ★ ★ ★
> TRAIL CONDITION: ★ ★ ★ ★
> CHILDREN: ★ ★ ★
> DIFFICULTY: ★
> SOLITUDE: ★ ★ ★ ★ ★

GPS TRAILHEAD COORDINATES: N33° 31.547' W86° 48.925'

DISTANCE & CONFIGURATION: 0.7-mile loop

HIKING TIME: If you really want to explore, allocate at least an hour.

HIGHLIGHTS: The final resting place of city pioneers, black and white; lovely statuary; peaceful atmosphere; beautiful trees; great views of the city skyline

ELEVATION: 615' at start, 705' at peak

ACCESS: Monday–Friday, 8 a.m.–4 p.m.

MAPS: Available at the cemetery office

FACILITIES: None

WHEELCHAIR ACCESS: Yes

COMMENTS: Be respectful. Don't touch the monuments. Pets are allowed on a leash, but you're asked to pick up after them.

CONTACT: Oak Hill Memorial Association, 205-251-6532, **oakhillbirmingham.com.**
The association sponsors seasonal tours.

Oak Hill Cemetery

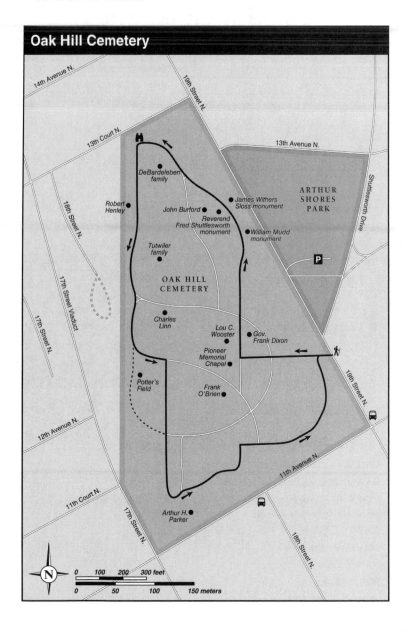

14th Avenue N.

19th Street N.

13th Court N.

13th Avenue N.

Shuttlesworth Drive

ARTHUR
SHORES
PARK

DeBardeleben
family

James Withers
Sloss monument

Robert
Henley

18th Street N.

John Burford

Reverend
Fred Shuttlesworth
monument

William Mudd
monument

P

Tutwiler
family

17th Street Viaduct

OAK HILL
CEMETERY

17th Street N.

Charles
Linn

Lou C.
Wooster

Gov.
Frank Dixon

Pioneer
Memorial
Chapel

19th Street N.

Potter's
Field

Frank
O'Brien

12th Avenue N.

11th Avenue N.

11th Court N.

17th Street N.

Arthur H.
Parker

18th Street N.

N

0   100   200   300 feet

0   50   100   150 meters

30

Overview

Madams and mayors, a soldier of the American Revolution and a leader of the civil rights movement, plantation owners and industrialists, victims of riots and murder and cholera, all resting in peace in a beautiful spot overlooking the city they shaped. A cemetery may seem an unlikely place for a hike, but you could spend years here gathering the stories waiting to be told.

Route Details

Most people stay out of cemeteries. I frequent this one. I run at lunch with a group of friends, and when we're feeling particularly lively, we loop through Oak Hill, which lies just west of the Birmingham-Jefferson Convention Complex.

Modern cemeteries are mostly austere and spare places. But Oak Hill, founded in 1871, in the earliest days of the city, is a romantic celebration of death.

Grand monuments and fine statuary, magnolias and oaks grace the winding walkways that mount a hillside. It can be a bear to run up on hot summer day. But once you crest that hill at the northern corner and begin your descent, you're rewarded with one of best views of city skyline. It's particularly pretty in the fall, with the leaves in full blaze, dying off for another winter. Those thoughts of mortality

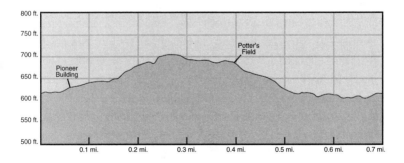

are all the more fitting as you're sharing your run with the ghosts of Birmingham past.

Nine of the 10 founders of Birmingham are buried here. One of the most recent additions is a principal founder of the new Birmingham: civil rights icon Fred Shuttlesworth.

It's a place full of juxtapositions, and it always has been. Many of the richest, most influential families are buried here, sharing the earth with the paupers buried without headstones in the cemetery's potter's field. Blacks and whites have been buried here in the same cemetery since its earliest days.

Enter the cemetery through the gates off 19th Street North and walk toward the **Pioneer Memorial Chapel,** the Tudor-style building that serves as the offices of the Oak Hill Memorial Association, the nonprofit organization entrusted since 1913 with the cemetery's care.

Start at the steps of that building and turn to your right, walking uphill. Just a few steps up the path, look to your left and you'll see a stone wall and some graves just above it. Search out the grave of **Louise Wooster** (1842–1913). Wooster was working as a prostitute in the fledging city when in 1873 cholera broke out. Half the city's 3,000 residents fled, but "Lou" was among those who stayed behind to nurture the sick and dying. According to legend, Wooster inspired the character Belle Watling in *Gone with the Wind.* (Margaret Mitchell lived briefly in Birmingham before writing the book.) Wooster, who claimed to have had a love affair with Abraham Lincoln's assassin, John Wilkes Booth, went on to operate a notorious brothel across the street from City Hall. It is said that though the respectable men of the town couldn't be seen attending her funeral, their empty, horse-drawn carriages formed a procession through Oak Hill in a show of respect at her passing. Inscribed on her tombstone: DEPARTED BUT NOT FORGOTTEN. For more of the fact and fiction of her life, read *A Woman of the Town,* by James Baggett, head of the Department of Archives and Manuscripts at the Birmingham Public Library.

Almost directly across the path from Wooster lies **Frank Dixon** (1892–1965). Governor of Alabama during the Depression and the

Second World War, Dixon was a progressive reformer who aggressively modernized state government. However, after leaving office, Dixon devoted himself to states' rights and rabid resistance to desegregation.

Continue straight, heading north and uphill. Look to the right and you'll see a couple of prominent obelisk-shaped monuments. The first honors **William Mudd** (1816–1884), a plantation owner and builder of Arlington, Birmingham's only antebellum plantation house. Shortly thereafter and also on the right side of the path is a monument to one of the founders of the post–Civil War industrial South, **James Withers Sloss** (1820–1890), who, as you might guess, built Sloss Furnaces, the former iron-making plant on First Avenue North right outside of downtown. And directly across the path from Sloss is a black granite memorial to the **Rev. Fred Shuttlesworth** (1922–2011), who more than anyone else deserves credit for leading the city to reinvent itself again. Coincidentally, the leader of Birmingham's civil rights movement grew up in Oxmoor Valley, not far from Birmingham's first iron ore mines and blast furnace. And maybe it's just another coincidence that the grave of **John Burford** (1758–1834), a veteran of the American War for Independence, is also buried nearby.

Continuing up the hill, on your left, you'll see the DeBardeleben family plot, where **Henry F. DeBardeleben** (1840–1910) and his wife, **Ellen Pratt DeBardeleben** (1844–1894), are buried. Ellen was the daughter of Daniel Pratt, considered Alabama's first industrialist, and Henry was a key player in launching Birmingham's industrial rise.

Rounding the crest of the cemetery hill and descending, you catch that view of the city I mentioned. To the left down the hill, in the shade of some of the cemetery's prettiest trees, is the **Tutwiler** family plot, a name associated with both the past of mining and industry and the development of downtown, including the Tutwiler Hotel, which was Birmingham's landmark hotel until its demolition in the 1970s. A former apartment building, also built by the Tutwilers, was later rechristened as the Tutwiler Hotel and still operates today.

33

As you come to an intersection with a path coming up the hill, take a detour down it and look for the mausoleum of banker and industrialist **Charles Linn** (1814–1882). A plaque on it bears a quote from Linn, made when Birmingham had a population of fewer than 4,000: "Bury me on the high promontory overlooking the city of Birmingham, in which you men profess to have little faith; so that I may walk out on Judgment Day and view the greatest industrial city in the entire South."

Return to the upper path. As you descend the upper ridge, you come to a wide, low open area in the southwest corner of the cemetery. Here lie the unmarked graves of the potter's field. Among those buried here are victims of the cholera epidemic. Also buried here are **Emma Hawes** (1859–1888) and her two daughters, victims of a grisly murder for which her husband, Richard, was convicted. Before the trial, a mob gathered at the courthouse where Richard Hawes was being held. As the mob advanced on the courthouse and failed to heed warnings to disperse, law-enforcement officers fired into the crowd, killing 10.

At the base of the hill, in the area around 11th Avenue North, you'll find the grave of **Arthur H. Parker** (1870–1939), the revered principal of Industrial High School for blacks, later renamed Parker High School in his honor. Also in this neighborhood is the grave of **William Pettiford** (1847–1914), whose Penny Savings Bank grew to be the largest and strongest African American–owned bank in the United States.

As you circle back toward the entrance, bear in mind that my listing only scratches the surface of the stories hidden here. You'll have to find on your own the graves of **Robert Henley,** the first mayor of Birmingham, and **Frank O'Brien,** the first mayor of Greater Birmingham, after the 1910 annexations that doubled the city's population.

Explore on your own. Maps are available at the cemetery office.

Directions

Oak Hill Cemetery is at the corner of 19th Street and 11th Avenue North, adjacent to the Birmingham-Jefferson Convention Complex.

3 # Railroad Park

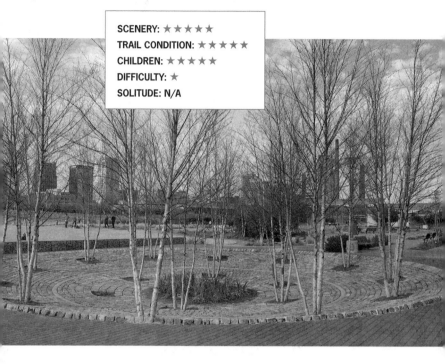

SCENERY: ★ ★ ★ ★ ★
TRAIL CONDITION: ★ ★ ★ ★ ★
CHILDREN: ★ ★ ★ ★ ★
DIFFICULTY: ★
SOLITUDE: N/A

GPS TRAILHEAD COORDINATES: N33° 30.611' W86° 48.506'

DISTANCE & CONFIGURATION: 1-mile loop

HIKING TIME: 30 minutes

HIGHLIGHTS: Open, urban hub for exercise and play; diverse and beautiful; mostly native landscaping; ponds and flowing creeks; 360-degree views of the skyline; city history exhibit; the motion, sound, and visual variety provided by passing trains

ELEVATION: Between 600' and 615'

ACCESS: Daily, 7 a.m.–11 p.m.

MAPS: Available at the website below

FACILITIES: Restrooms, concession stand, bike racks, picnic table, benches, playgrounds, exercise area, skateboard bowls, amphitheater

WHEELCHAIR ACCESS: Yes

COMMENTS: Pets welcome but must be under control and on a leash at all times, and you need to clean up after them. Bikers, skaters, and skateboarders are allowed but are asked to use the central paved corridor. Free Wi-Fi is available throughout the park.

CONTACT: 205-521-9933, **railroadpark.org**

Railroad Park

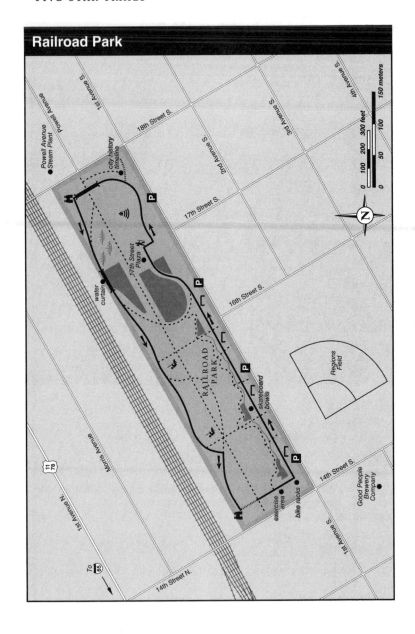

Overview

Railroad Park is ground zero for the new Birmingham, a recycled and resurgent city, a Birmingham of shared space. It's a center of activity where a diverse citizenry meets to relax or recreate. The park comprises four city blocks, 19 acres, with ponds and streams and native trees, flowers, and grasses. There are wide-open meadows and undulating hills. In the fall, hillsides of muhly grass turn a blazing pink, and in the summer, a profusion of flowers blooms. There are playgrounds and exercise equipment, dining on the plaza, and a grassy amphitheater for concerts. Elevated walkways allow you to survey the city center in every direction: the downtown skyline; trains rolling through the center of town; the city's new ballpark, Regions Field; the towers of Children's Hospital; the University of Alabama at Birmingham's medical complex and college campus; and Vulcan, atop Red Mountain.

Route Details

When the 21st century dawned, the four blocks that now make up Railroad Park were a forlorn, weed-choked lot that had once been a railroad freight yard. To the north, the office-oriented downtown was beginning to add more restaurants and living spaces. To the south, the medical and university district was seeing constant construction of new buildings and housing. The gathering momentum gave energy to an idea that had been dreamed about for decades: Take that neglected no-man's-land south of the downtown rail corridor and turn it into a ribbon of green running through the heart of the city. Create a place to play, to wander, to gather; a place for outdoor concerts and festivals; a place to exercise or relax.

Most older major cities grew up along rivers, and revitalization efforts have tended to center along their waterfronts, but Birmingham's river was the railroads. So we turned to the tracks.

The construction of the park was a partnership of many players, public and private. The nonprofit Railroad Park Foundation and the city of Birmingham led the way, with support from Jefferson County, the Community Foundation of Greater Birmingham, and a multitude of other donors. The park cost $23 million to build and opened in 2010 to immediate success, followed by a long list of awards and recognitions. It spurred the construction of Regions Field across First Avenue South from the park. It has also inspired residential projects in the area and the development of greenways and trails spreading out from the park in every direction.

Start your walk at the 17th Street Plaza, north of the intersection of 17th Street South and First Avenue South. This plaza serves as the main hub of the park, where you can find the park headquarters, restrooms, and a concession area.

From the plaza, proceed east, uphill on the asphalt walkway that ascends the southern edge of the big grassy bowl. You're walking parallel to First Avenue South. As you climb this hill, it's a good moment to observe how the park's designers reshaped the landscape for both aesthetic and functional purposes. Before the park, this was a flat plain, the lowest point in the city. It was bounded in the north by a tall, unsightly wall rising to the railroad corridor.

During the construction process, the land was reconfigured to form this amphitheater to host concerts and movies. They dug out the ponds and piled up earth to create a hillside along the northern edge of the park. That landscaped hillside now hides the viaduct wall, and its upper ridge carries an elevated walkway from which you can view the city, the park, and the rolling rail corridor.

As you reach the top of the amphitheater knoll, a brick staircase descends to the corner of 18th Street South and First Avenue South. Along this staircase is a timeline display of the city's history. Take a detour to explore it, but be careful not to get so wrapped up in the story that you stumble down the steps.

Continuing on the elevated walk, cross a bridge above the park's central paved corridor, an extension of Powell Avenue through the park. Proceeding to the far northeast corner of the park, you arrive at a viewing platform situated at the park's highest point.

This is the best spot to take in the view of the entire park and the surrounding city. From this vantage point, you can connect the origins of the city with its present. The rail corridor before you was the reason the city grew in the spot that it did. From this juncture, train routes coming in from the north, south, east, and west converge.

The earliest iron furnaces in the city—Sloss Furnaces, still visible to the east, and the Alice Furnace, which was a few blocks west of the park's western end—were built on this corridor. Locally mined iron ore, coal, and limestone flowed into those furnaces from the surrounding countryside by rail.

Directly across 18th Street South is a large brick building, which until recently was a coal-fired steam plant that once generated electricity for an extensive streetcar system centered here. It also provided steam heat for the city's progression of rising office buildings clustered along 20th Street South to the north of the rail corridor.

Looking back to the park, you can pick out the subtle ways designers used native elements in creating the landscape: brick made from our red-clay soils, limestone collected in metal cages to form much of the bench seating. Steel bridges and structures suggest our steel industry. The buildings on the plaza call to mind railroad boxcars.

The park's hillsides, planted with native grasses, flowers, and trees, slope down to the water features that collect storm water and recirculate it through the park. A wetland marsh of cattails and aquatic grasses and flowers at the eastern end of the park serves as a biofiltration system. The collected water is supplemented with water drawn from on-site wells and is used to irrigate the park. The park's four square blocks have been sculpted into a microcosm of the region, with its valleys, ridges, creeks, and wetlands.

Proceeding to the west, you stay at the level of the trains, which, as they clank and grind through town, create an ever-changing display of movement, sight, and sound. You cross above a rain curtain that drops into a pond. In the pond, you might spot carp released to control vegetation, along with little swarms of goldfish that seem to have been an unsanctioned addition.

The trail dips down off the ridge, passing close to a children's playground, then rises again to the northwest corner of the park. An observation platform here provides a view of Regions Field, home of the Birmingham Barons, the city's longtime minor-league baseball team. The Barons moved from their original home at Rickwood Field to a suburban park in Hoover in 1988, but they returned to the central city 25 years later. Named the nation's best new ballpark of 2013, Regions Field drew huge crowds in its inaugural season. If you haven't been to a game, you're missing out. Get down there.

Descend the stairs and continue parallel to 14th Street South, crossing the Powell Avenue corridor, then passing an area devoted to exercise equipment. As you reach the southwest corner of the park and start heading back toward the entry plaza, you have a choice of three distinct corridors: a paved path for runners and walkers, a gravel promenade for ambling and pausing to enjoy the scenery, and a streetside brick sidewalk. The paved track runs along a curving creek bed whose banks are formed by granite street curbs salvaged during the park's excavation.

The gravel promenade is punctuated by flower beds and passes through two smaller entrance plazas. At the 15th Street South plaza, you can pause to watch skateboarders dipping, swooping, and speeding along the contours of three skate bowls. The 16th Street South plaza centers on a small grove of river birch trees, planted in a dug-out bowl surfaced with cobblestones unearthed during the park's construction.

As you proceed back toward the entrance plaza, you'll also note the cobblestones used to line the banks of a smaller pond adjacent to the plaza.

If you're determined to keep walking, you can recirculate along the gravel path that winds along the course of the creek and mix and match other paths.

However, one of the real pleasures of the park is sitting on a bench or on the grass and watching the swirl of humanity. All ages and races share this space.

No place where people gather is completely immune to conflict and tension, but Railroad Park is remarkable for its daily production of positive energy and interaction among its diverse clientele. It's a civic space that Birmingham, in particular, has long needed. And discovering that has been a huge boost to the spirit of the city.

Nearby Attractions

Regions Field, home of the Birmingham Barons, is at the corner of 14th Street and First Avenue South, right across from the park (205-988-3200, **tinyurl.com/regionsfield**). Half a block south of that corner, at 114 14th St. S., is the **Good People Brewing Company** (205-286-2337, **goodpeoplebrewing.com**). The taproom is open every afternoon and into the evening. Brewery tours (reservations suggested) are available on Saturdays, 2–4 p.m. You might also want to combine a visit to Railroad Park with a stop at **McWane Science Center,** at 200 19th St. N. (see page 21), featuring IMAX movies, interactive exhibits, dinosaurs, aquariums, and a whole lot more. **Sloss Furnaces,** at 20 32nd St. N., offers self-guided and scheduled guided tours of the historic iron-making blast furnaces that helped build the city (205-324-1911, **slossfurnaces.com**). And the **Alabama Theatre** (see page 21), the gloriously restored movie palace at 1817 Third Ave. N., offers summer and holiday film series.

Directions

Railroad Park is on First Avenue South in downtown Birmingham, between 14th and 18th Streets South. Street parking is available on First Avenue South and the surrounding blocks. Park patrons are also welcome to use the Birmingham Parking Authority's Lot D, on 18th Street South and First Avenue South, at a cost of $2.

Vulcan Trail–
Southside Loop

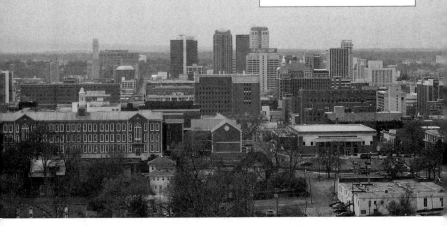

SCENERY: ★ ★ ★ ★ ★
TRAIL CONDITION: ★ ★ ★ ★
CHILDREN: ★ ★ ★
DIFFICULTY: ★ ★ ★
SOLITUDE: ★

GPS TRAILHEAD COORDINATES: N33° 29.556′ W86° 47.730′

DISTANCE & CONFIGURATION: 4.1-mile loop

HIKING TIME: Budget half a day for this adventure.

HIGHLIGHTS: Vulcan, the world's largest cast-iron statue; views of the city from Vulcan Trail; the University of Alabama at Birmingham; Five Points South (restaurants, shops, Five Points fountain, and Brother Bryan statue); Cobb Lane

ELEVATION: 911′ at trailhead, 610′ at lowest point

ACCESS: Vulcan Park is open Monday–Saturday, 10 a.m.–6 p.m., and Sunday, 1–6 p.m. The observation tower stays open until 10 p.m. Admission is $6 for adults, $5 for seniors age 65 and over and for military, and $4 for children ages 5–12. Children age 4 and under are admitted free. After 6 p.m., admission is $4 for adults age 5 and up.

MAPS: A street map of Birmingham might come in handy.

FACILITIES: Vulcan Park has restrooms, picnic tables, and water fountains.

WHEELCHAIR ACCESS: Vulcan Park and Vulcan Trail are wheelchair-accessible. The rest of the route is accessible to the extent that urban environments are accessible. The one stretch that is definitely *not* accessible is the sidewalk going up Red Mountain along 20th Street South and Richard Arrington Jr. Boulevard South: It's barely passable for pedestrians, difficult for anyone walking a bike, and, I would think, totally out of the question for wheelchair access considering the light and power poles planted in the narrow sidewalk.

COMMENTS: Aside from the final climb back up Red Mountain, this makes a great bike ride. Consider riding and then locking up your bike at the base of the mountain for pickup later. This ride goes through an urban environment, so be prepared for lively, pleasant activity, along with challenges from traffic to panhandling.

CONTACT: Vulcan Park & Museum, 205-933-1409, **visitvulcan.com**

Overview

This hike hits highlights of Birmingham past and future, starting with the world's largest cast-iron statue, Vulcan, the Roman god of the forge, erected in tribute to the iron and steel industries that built Birmingham. The hike proceeds along a section of what used to be the Birmingham Mineral Railroad, which once served the mines along the mountainside and is now a paved greenway with views of the city skyline. The walk then descends into the new center of Birmingham's economy, the University of Alabama at Birmingham. After ambling through the campus, we head to the dining and entertainment district at Five Points South and up quaint Cobb Lane. Finally, we make a steep ascent along 20th Street South back to the Vulcan Trail parking lot.

Route Details

Birmingham is becoming a more welcoming place for walking and biking, but the beginning and end of this route point to work still left to be done.

If you plan to incorporate a visit to **Vulcan Park & Museum** into this hike (and you should if you haven't been in a while), you'll need to drive to the park to enjoy the excellent museum and beautiful grounds, ride up the glass elevator to the statue's observation deck, and get a great view of the city.

Then you'll need to get back in your car and drive to the separate parking lot for Vulcan Trail, off Richard Arrington Jr. Boulevard South and just north of Vulcan Park, on the Birmingham side of the mountain.

43

Vulcan Trail–Southside Loop

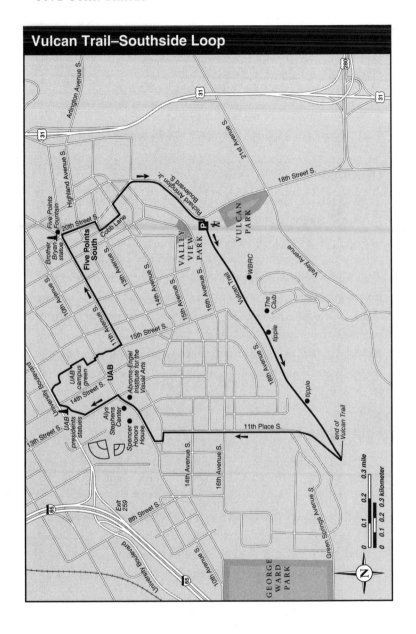

Take care turning into this parking lot if you're coming up the mountain from Vulcan Park. It may be safer to drive over the mountain and come back up 20th Street South so you can make a right turn into the parking lot. Also, bear in mind that this lot can fill up on a sunny day.

One day, hopefully, the park and the trail will be reconnected; they were historically. Vulcan sits atop the Valley View Mine (1904–1924), and the Vulcan Trail follows the bed of the railroad that picked up ore at this mine and numerous others from Ruffner Mountain to Bessemer.

Start by following the path from the parking lot back up to the fence that serves as the boundary to Vulcan Park. Between the grounds around the statue and the trail is an unrestored area of original stonework, courtesy of the Civilian Conservation Corps, the men put back to work during the Depression. The CCC laid the foundation for this park and numerous others.

Proceed west on this smooth paved surface (it's a nice route on a bike as well). Looking up the kudzu-covered mountain slope, you'll see two of the local television stations, **WVTM** (NBC 13) and **WBRC** (Fox 6), high atop the mountain. WBRC has a distinctive red neon sign. (The last three call letters stand for "Bell Radio Corporation"; J. C. Bell founded the station's radio predecessor in the 1920s.) Also perched on the mountain is **The Club,** a swanky jet-age supper club.

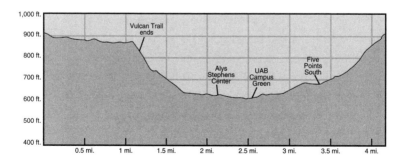

45

Turn your attention to the valley below for wide-open views of UAB and the city skyline. On a clear day, you can see on the north-western horizon the steam rising from Alabama Power's Miller Electric Generating Plant. The trail is a heck of a place to catch a sunset, but it isn't lit, so I wouldn't linger.

Just past The Club you'll see the base of what was a tipple, one of two along this stretch. These were the structures where the iron ore brought up from the mines was loaded into train cars.

Incidentally, the kudzu covering these slopes is also a remnant of the mining operations. Kudzu was promoted as an excellent erosion-preventer and was often planted at former mine sites to stabilize the hillsides. This was in the days before companies were required to reclaim the disturbed land. As you proceed farther, you'll notice the much more appealing natural vegetation. Oakleaf hydrangea in particular is a beautiful and tenacious comeback kid along these ridges.

The Vulcan Trail officially ends at 1.2 miles. A gated paved road leads up the hill to Water Works tanks, and an unsanctioned dirt trail heads off into the underbrush. Hopefully, one day the trail will extend all the way to Green Springs Avenue along this same railroad bed. Using street connections from there, Vulcan Park could tie into Red Mountain Park.

But for now we're headed into the city, down the steep hill to join 11th Place South. Take this road straight, through a funky neighborhood of older homes. Some have been restored and look great, and others are occupied by college students. Coming down this street, there is a great moment when the city skyline comes into view.

After you pass Glen Iris Elementary School, follow the road as it curves to a stoplight at 10th Avenue South. Take a right there or, if you choose, use the crosswalk to cross to the opposite side of the street and onto the **UAB** campus.

Proceed east on 10th Avenue, and on your right you'll see what used to be Second Presbyterian Church but now is the home of UAB's honors program, the **Spencer Honors House** (no relation to me).

Just beyond that is the **Alys Stephens Performing Arts Center,** a venue for concerts and plays. Across the street is one of the newest buildings on the UAB campus, the **Abroms-Engel Institute for the Visual Arts,** which includes art galleries open weekdays, 10 a.m.–6 p.m., and Saturday, noon–6 p.m.

At the next corner, at 10th Avenue and 13th Street South, turn left and proceed north on 13th Street to University Boulevard. Cross 13th Street, heading east into a small park planted with live oaks and cherry blossom trees.

Near the easternmost corner of this park are statues of the first three presidents of UAB: Joseph Volker, S. Richardson Hill, and Charles "Scotty" McCallum. Volker arrived at UAB in 1945, when the school was simply an extension of the mother campus in Tuscaloosa. He was the key leader in the rapid development of UAB into a top-tier medical-research university. He became its first president, serving from 1969 to 1976. His statue is flanked by those of his two successors, Hill and McCallum, who carried on Volker's work. Under subsequent presidents, J. Claude Bennett, Ann Reynolds, Carol Garrison, and the current president, Ray Watts, UAB has continued to expand its research base but has also become a more traditional undergraduate college.

That's evident on the next block, where there is now a sprawling campus green. As of 2014, a new student center was under construction across University Boulevard, and the green itself had just gained a dragon, UAB's mascot rendered in topiary.

Proceed south through the green back toward Red Mountain, taking in the sights. Cross 10th Avenue South and follow the pedestrian path at the center of the block through the dorms and 11th Avenue South. Here, take a left and proceed east toward 20th Street South. After four blocks, you enter the **Five Points South** district. You have a multitude of places to eat or drink here, including Frank Stitt's nationally known fine-dining restaurant, **Highlands Bar and Grill,** and its casual cousin, **Chez Fonfon.** For vegetarians, **Golden Temple** is a

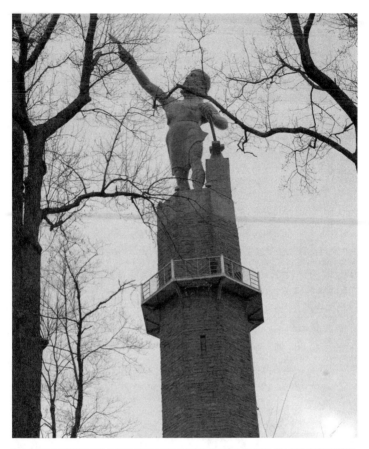

VULCAN SURVEYS HIS DOMAIN FROM HIS RENOVATED PERCH ON RED MOUNTAIN.

Birmingham institution, and across 11th Avenue South, there's barbecue at **Jim 'N Nicks** and Thai food at **Surin West.** I could go on.

Music fans might want to wander upstairs to **Charlemagne Records** or across 20th Street to **Renaissance Records.** On the way, see the **Five Points Fountain** and its whimsical statues created by Birmingham artist Frank Fleming. On a corner adjacent to the Five Points intersection is a statue of **James A. Bryan,** pastor of Third Presbyterian Church from 1889 to 1941. "Brother Bryan" was famous for his tireless ministry to Birmingham's homeless.

Proceed south on 20th Street up the mountain, past additional dining and drinking options. At the corner of 20th Street and 13th Avenue South, take a right and then look to the left for a redbrick alley, Cobb Lane. Enjoy a stroll up the quaint lane, and if you're so inclined, stop to wet your whistle at **The J. Clyde,** a restaurant and bar with an unrivaled selection of beers. There is a parking lot at the uphill end of Cobb Lane. If you rode a bike, you might want to lock it up here—it's a steep and dangerous climb beyond this point.

You could also stop at **Valley View Park** on the way up. It's a slight diversion up 19th Street South. Valley View Park allows you to get up close to what used to be a mine entrance. However, when we visited, there was some sketchy activity, and I felt like we were walking through someone's living area.

Regardless, you can't avoid going back to 20th Street and ascending Red Mountain on some pretty cruddy sidewalks. It's a steep climb, but there is a great moment at the end, when you've gotten back close to the top and can look out over the city again.

Directions

Coming from the Birmingham side of the mountain, drive up 20th Street and look for the signs to Vulcan Trail. If you want to start at Vulcan Park, continue past the Vulcan Trail parking lot and take your next right, a sharp turn back up the mountain and up to Vulcan. If you're coming up the mountain heading to the Vulcan Trail from Homewood and points south, parking for the trail is just after you crest the mountain. Turn left into the parking lot, but be careful: The road down the mountain makes a sharp curve, and it's hard to see cars speeding up the mountain.

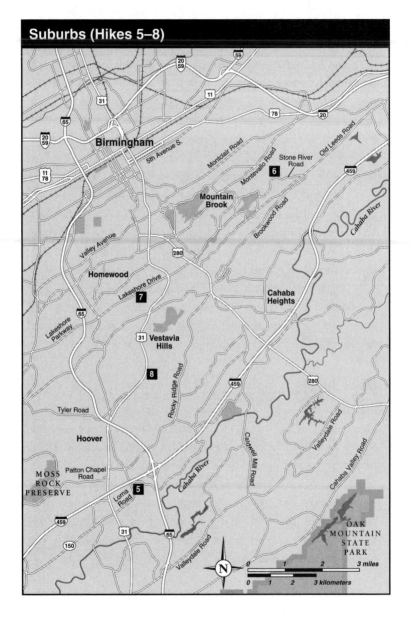

Suburbs (Hikes 5–8)

Birmingham

20 59
59
11
31
65
20 59
11 78

5th Avenue S.
Montclair Road
Montevallo Road
Stone River Road
Old Leeds Road
78
20
6
459

Mountain Brook

Valley Avenue

Homewood

Lakeshore Drive
7

280

Cahaba Heights

Cahaba River

65

Lakeshore Parkway

31 Vestavia Hills

8

Rocky Ridge Road

459

280

Tyler Road

Hoover

MOSS ROCK PRESERVE

Patton Chapel Road

Lorna Road

5

Cahaba River

Caldwell Mill Road

Valleydale Road

Cahaba Valley Road

459

150

31

65

Valleydale Road

OAK MOUNTAIN STATE PARK

N

0   1   2   3 miles

0   1   2   3 kilometers

Suburbs

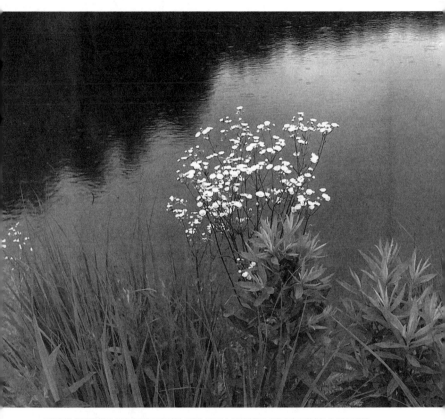

QUEEN ANNE'S LACE BLOOMS ALONG THE LAKESIDE AT ALDRIDGE GARDENS IN HOOVER. *(See Hike 5.)*

Suburbs Overview

After treating walking as an afterthought in most developments in the second half of the 20th century, the suburbs have rediscovered the importance of including accommodations for pedestrians.

Mountain Brook led the way in this movement. A greenway built through Jemison Park along Shades Creek and Mountain Brook Parkway brought people out to enjoy that little chunk of woods in the midst of suburbia. That was just the beginning of a movement for greenways and sidewalks that now stretch throughout that city.

Homewood joined in with the construction of the Shades Creek Greenway and the preservation of the Homewood Forest Preserve. Despite its beautiful but challenging topography, **Vestavia Hills** has been investing in sidewalks. And when it came time to build a new library, they perched it on the edge of the forest, creating a one-stop destination for reading and a walk in the woods.

Meanwhile, Irondale and Trussville have both launched greenway projects along the Cahaba River, and a coalition of communities north of Birmingham is working to develop a long-distance greenway along Five Mile Creek.

With Ruffner Mountain Nature Preserve, Oak Mountain State Park, Red Mountain Park, and Moss Rock Preserve, we're lucky to have major go-to venues for hiking, but it has been gratifying to see further development of trails embedded in the fabric of communities. The **Freshwater Land Trust (freshwaterlandtrust.org)** led the development of a regional master plan consisting of hundreds of miles of potential trails and sidewalks. If you like the concept of in-town hiking, the **Red Rock Ridge & Valley Trail System (redrocktrail.org)** is a good place to find a project you can support.

Even in built-out urban and suburban environments, it's amazing to see what creativity and community willpower can bring about. All about the region there are stream corridors, old railroad beds, and utility easements that can be repurposed for trails where there are willing neighbors and a community desire to make it happen.

Aldridge Gardens

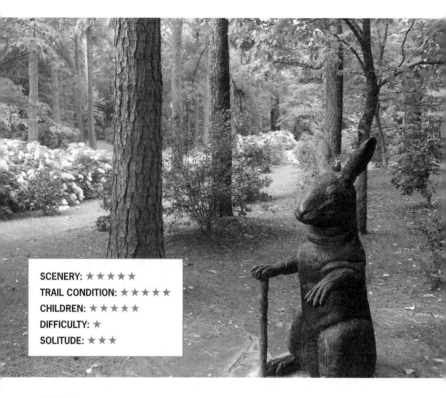

SCENERY: ★ ★ ★ ★ ★
TRAIL CONDITION: ★ ★ ★ ★ ★
CHILDREN: ★ ★ ★ ★ ★
DIFFICULTY: ★
SOLITUDE: ★ ★ ★

GPS TRAILHEAD COORDINATES: N33° 23.206' W86° 47.616'

DISTANCE & CONFIGURATION: 1-mile loop

HIKING TIME: 1 hour

HIGHLIGHTS: A peaceful pond; tall pines; wandering waterfowl; whimsical statues; magnolias, ferns, and flowers; but most particularly and most abundantly, hydrangeas—hydrangeas of every kind

ELEVATION: 516' at the start, 535' at the peak, 483' at the low point

ACCESS: Daily, 8 a.m.–5 p.m. Admission is free.

MAPS: Available at the entrance gate and the website below

FACILITIES: Restrooms, pavilion, picnic tables, benches, gift shop

WHEELCHAIR ACCESS: Yes

COMMENTS: No pets allowed

CONTACT: 205-682-8019, **aldridgegardens.com**

Aldridge Gardens

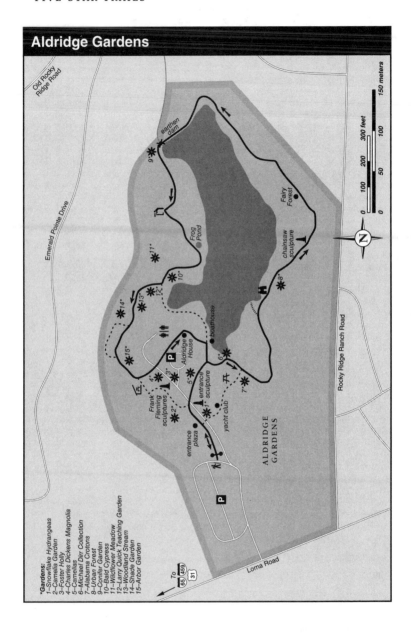

Gardens:
1—Snowflake Hydrangeas
2—Camelia Garden
3—Foster Holly
4—Charles Dickens Magnolia
5—Camelias
6—Michael Dirr Collection
7—Alabama Crotons
8—Urban Forest
9—Conifer Garden
10—Bald Cypress
11—Wildflower Meadow
12—Larry Quick Teaching Garden
13—Woodland Stream
14—Shade Garden
15—Arbor Garden

ALDRIDGE GARDENS

Overview

Opened in 2002, this 30-acre botanical garden owned by the city of Hoover was once the home of Eddie and Kay Aldridge. Eddie and his father owned a plant nursery and were particularly renowned for patenting and propagating the snowflake hydrangea, an elegant double-blooming variant of the oakleaf hydrangea. Snowflake hydrangeas are plentiful here, along with numerous other hydrangea varieties, as well as a diverse offering of other flowers, trees, and scenery. An easy, scenic hike around the park's 5-acre lake gives a little dose of piney woodlands, wildflowers, and still waters. Along the way, you're likely to meet families of ducks and geese. Follow that with an exploration of the house, its sunny landscaped grounds, and a maze of shady gardens nearby.

Route Details

The oakleaf hydrangea was designated Alabama's state wildflower in 1999, in long overdue recognition of the faithful, hardy decorator of Alabama forests. On many of the hikes in this book, hydrangeas are a key ingredient in the mix that makes a beautiful landscape. At Aldridge Gardens, they take center stage.

Our native hydrangeas are sometimes neglected in favor of the showy pink and blue French hydrangeas that are a favorite element in Southern gardening. Eddie Aldridge, a nursery owner and the father of Aldridge Gardens, deserves much credit for putting our native hydrangeas on the equal footing they should enjoy. Long before the modern native-plant craze, Aldridge celebrated the oakleaf, which loves shade and moist soil but can withstand heat and drought.

In its typical form, the oakleaf is subtly beautiful, with its fresh green growth in spring, its clouds of creamy white blooms in early summer, and its rusty red coloring in the fall. Aldridge popularized a variant of the oakleaf, the snowflake, which in effect has double the blooms of a normal oakleaf. The original plant was found in the wild around Turkey Creek in Pinson. When a customer brought in a cutting, the Aldridges realized it was special, propagated it, and, in 1971, patented it. Eddie is also credited with helping introduce the 'Harmony' hydrangea, which was discovered growing on the grounds of Harmony Baptist Church in Attalla. The 'Harmony' produces a big, billowing blob of a bloom, packed with thousands of tiny white flowers.

Both varieties are on display in the entrance plaza of the gardens, where this hike begins. The plaza's focal point is *On the Nature of Building,* by sculptor Ted Metz. That urnlike shape hanging from a cable in the center of the sculpture is a plumb bob, a tool used since ancient times that helps builders determine whether what they are building is in vertical alignment. At the base of that are other instruments used in design, along with a small bird with a twig for its nest in its mouth. It's a good place to think about how the garden is a collaboration between nature's creation and the gentle guiding hand of humans.

Branching off to the right of the entrance plaza is a path to a picnic area shaded by tall pines, dogwoods, and magnolias and ringed by an understory of azaleas and French blue hydrangeas. You can immediately set off through the picnic area for a loop around the lake, but to take an initial taste of the garden, I'd advise walking forward a bit. On your left, to the north of the entry plaza, is a collection of camellias. Though it is native to Japan, China, and other Asian countries, the *Camellia japonica* became Alabama's state flower in 1960. Give camellias their due: They are beautiful, various, and a staple of Southern gardens. Forty varieties can be found in this collection.

Just beyond the camellia gardens are two sculptures by beloved Birmingham artist Frank Fleming. *Along for the Ride* features a tortoise pulling a cart in which a hare is riding. Nearby, another Fleming-sculpted bunny is *Waiting for My Ride.* You can see more of Fleming's sculptures in the fountain at Five Points South and around the grounds of the Birmingham Botanical Gardens. Fleming's work gets you in the mood to put a little more imagination into the walk you're about to enjoy.

From here, you can get a glimpse of the house and gardens overlooking the lake. Bear right toward the lake, following the path into a low area near the lake's boathouse, and find the path that leads toward the southern shore of the lake. I prefer to make this circuit around the lake before enjoying the more manicured gardens around the house.

Find the sign for the lake trail, which takes you up the ridge a bit before dropping back down to the lakeside. This walk features oakleaf hydrangeas under the canopy of forest with nice views of the green lake below. It must be said that with I-459 just to the north and I-65 just to the east, there's no escaping the muffled rumble of traffic.

You'll reach a trail junction marked by a sculpture of a crowned and bearded king carved with a chainsaw from a tree trunk. You have a choice here of taking the high road through the Fairy Forest or sticking to the low road by the lake. The Fairy Forest features a little natural playground equipped with sticks and stones and pinecones children use to create miniature landscapes for forest dwellers.

The high trail descends and intersects with the low trail and continues the circuit around the lake by crossing the dam at the far end of the lake. It's a nice vantage point and in the summer it's covered with Queen Anne's lace. The trail crosses a bridge over the dam's spillway and continues through a strip of woods between the lake and an open, sunny corridor of low vegetation. Birds are abundant in this borderland and an Eagle Scout–built observation deck provides a nice spot to look and listen.

Continuing around the lake, the path takes you by a lakeside pair of bronze frog sculptures. Ahead is a wildflower meadow, which marks the entrance to a series of gardens to the rear of the house. The shady gardens have more varieties of hydrangea, plus ferns and hostas. You can usually find a spot to sit alone back here and enjoy the sound of water flowing through an artfully constructed water feature.

The winding path next leads to the arbor garden, a grassy lawn enclosed by a border of 'Annabelle' hydrangeas (also a native variety), ferns, and azaleas, as well as pines and magnolias. It's a favorite spot for weddings and makes a nice picnic area too.

Arriving back at the house, you can tour its art gallery, which is open on weekdays. Don't forget to come around to the front of the house. In the sunny lawn overlooking the lake, I found a rainbow assortment of daylilies in bloom as well as other colorful ornamentals mixed into a bed at the feet of a St. Francis of Assisi statue. You might want to make a final stop at the boathouse, which has been converted into a covered picnic area.

From that lakefront, looking back at the house and grounds and the surrounding gardens, I felt a real appreciation for the effort and eye that went into sculpting the place and a real thankfulness that Aldridge, Hoover, and a deep bench of volunteers have made available this oasis in the midst of Hoover's rapid growth.

Directions

From I-65, take Exit 252, where I-65 and US 31 meet between Hoover and Vestavia Hills; Lorna Road branches off US 31 just south of that exit. Follow Lorna Road to Aldridge Gardens, at 3530 Lorna Road, 2 miles ahead on your left after you cross over I-459. Coming from the other direction, AL 150 in Hoover becomes Lorna Road east of its intersection with US 31 near the Riverchase Galleria.

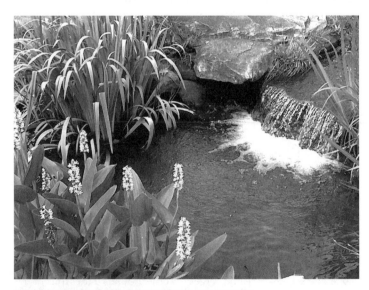

A WATER FEATURE FLOWS PAST GRASSES AND BLOOMS.

Irondale Furnace & Mountain Brook Trails

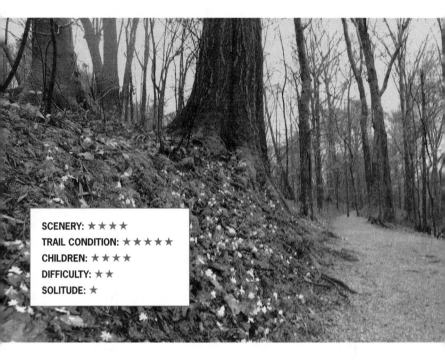

SCENERY: ★ ★ ★ ★
TRAIL CONDITION: ★ ★ ★ ★ ★
CHILDREN: ★ ★ ★ ★
DIFFICULTY: ★ ★
SOLITUDE: ★

GPS TRAILHEAD COORDINATES: N33° 30.414' W86° 43.596'

DISTANCE & CONFIGURATION: 4.5-mile point-to-point; requires a shuttle

HIKING TIME: 3 hours

HIGHLIGHTS: Historic ironworks ruins, Shades Creek, beautiful homes with landscaped yards

ELEVATION: 670' at start, 807' at peak

ACCESS: Daily; no charge

MAPS: A map of trails and sidewalks in the city is available on the "Parks and Trails" page of the website below.

FACILITIES: Benches throughout, picnic tables in Jemison Park, dog-waste disposal bags at strategic spots

WHEELCHAIR ACCESS: The trail to Irondale Furnace should pose no problem.

COMMENTS: After a heavy rain, the Shades Creek crossing on Jemison Trail just west of Overbrook Road will be submerged and impassable.

CONTACT: Mountain Brook Parks and Recreation, 205-802-3877, **mtnbrook.org**

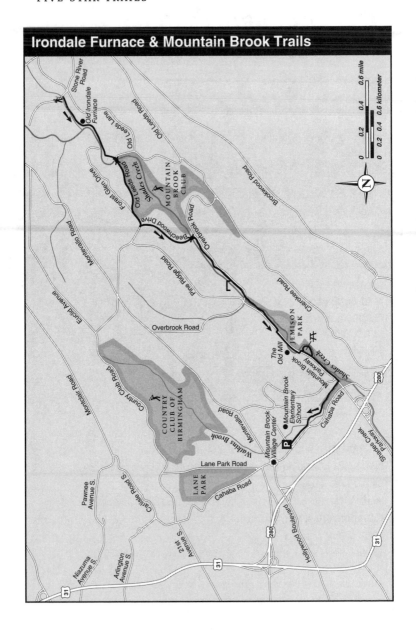

Irondale Furnace & Mountain Brook Trails

Overview

This hike takes you from a Civil War–era iron furnace through one of the finest suburban developments of the 20th century to a commercial village in the midst of a 21st-century update. You'll not only see landscaped yards stocked with imported Southern classics like camellias, azaleas, and cherry trees, but you'll also enjoy natural areas with unexpected native botanical variety. Grand homes are on display throughout. They come in a variety of sizes and styles, but they're consistently attractive and well cared for.

This hike could be broken into several out-and-backs. You have several places to park and pick up the route.

Route Details

This hike is a bit of an odyssey, but it's worth a little logistical maneuvering. Start by dropping a car in Mountain Brook Village in order to have a shuttle back to the start. The athletic fields at Mountain Brook Elementary, at the intersection of Cahaba Road and Heathermoor Road, might be a good place to park.

Look around in the village and enjoy your drive to the trailhead. I grew up in Mountain Brook, but revisiting this route has again deepened my appreciation for its original vision and the continued cultivation and extension of those ideas.

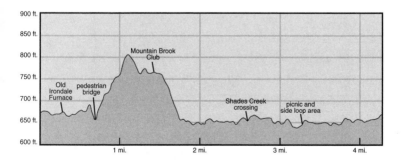

The story told on this hike begins long before the city of Mountain Brook was conceived. On the way to the trailhead, drive out Montevallo Road and note a historical marker beside a log structure visible from the road. It's near the corner of Montevallo Road and Glenbrook Drive.

This cabin was originally built in the 1820s, part of the earliest wave of settlement in the area after Andrew Jackson's campaign against the Creek Indians during the War of 1812. I grew up a stone's throw away from here and have driven on Montevallo Road all my life without appreciating that it was one of the early principal routes through the area.

In the 1860s, that cabin and its additions were repurposed to serve as the commissary for the industrial operation at the Irondale Furnace, where we begin this hike.

Until recently, the stone ruins of the Confederate-era ironworks were hidden by privet in a little patch of no-man's-land forest in Mountain Brook's Cherokee Bend neighborhood. Now, the privet has been cleared, the trails improved, and interpretive signage installed.

In the 1860s, the Irondale Furnace operation covered a huge expanse, from well south of this site on the creek up to Red Mountain and the iron ore mines there. The furnace was fired by timber cut from the more than 2,000 acres surrounding it. The pig iron was then sent by oxcart down Montevallo Road to Montevallo, where it was loaded on trains bound for the Confederate arsenal at Selma. In 1865, Union soldiers likely traveled Montevallo Road on their way to burn the ironworks. (I had always wondered why all the roads in Cherokee Bend were named for Confederate battles. I guess the developer was harking back to this Civil War connection.)

To begin the hike, park across from the historical marker at Stone River Road and follow the gravel path beside Furnace Creek about 0.3 mile to the site. You'll find tall stone walls built into a hillside. The interpretive signage helps you picture what the furnace operation looked like. There are benches and open green space. If you just want a short walk and a picnic, you can stop here.

But for the extended tour, we'll continue on the gravel path beyond the furnace ruins out to Shades Creek. This modest-sized creek obviously drew early activity from this furnace to one several miles downstream near Bluff Park, where another Civil War furnace, the Oxmoor Furnace, was built.

And the founders of Mountain "Brook" saw the waterway as an attractive asset. As you'll see as we proceed, the creek flows through Mountain Brook Club's golf course and runs alongside Mountain Brook Parkway.

Shades Creek can be lovely, but don't expect something pristine. When the water rises, it turns milk-chocolate brown, and plastic shopping bags and other debris are left stranded in the tree limbs. Perhaps we'll figure out how to keep the bottles and balls, tires and other trash from ending up in our streams, but for now we take the bad with the good.

Leaving the furnace site, you'll see some nice native vegetation along the trail. Oakleaf hydrangeas and mountain laurels bloom in late spring and summer.

On the opposite bank of the creek, you can see houses at the end of Forest Glen Drive. The trail winds for about 0.3 mile until it intersects a paved driveway—take a right and continue out to Old Leeds Road. At Old Leeds, turn right and cross a new pedestrian bridge over Shades Creek. From it, you can view a set of shoals upstream in the creek. Looking downstream, also note the stonework on the road bridge. You'll see this native sandstone again and again; it was used throughout the original Mountain Brook development in the 1920s. Beyond the bridge, you can see the Mountain Brook Club golf course spreading out across the floodplain, cupped by low surrounding ridges.

Proceed up the hill along the sidewalk, looking out for the nice landscaping along the way. At the top of the hill, you'll cross Forest Glen Drive and take your next left onto Beechwood Drive. To be safe, however, proceed to the crosswalk at the next intersection, then walk back up to Beechwood.

As you head down the Beechwood hill, on your left you get a glimpse of Mountain Brook Club, a private country club. The white-columned clubhouse is visible through a scattering of tall pine trees and magnolias.

On your right, across the street, houses are perched along a small ridge. The city's planners picked each home site carefully, after an extensive survey of the existing terrain. The houses were oriented to have a good view and yet have privacy from one another. You will also notice that the driveways of the houses are cut unobtrusively into the landscape. Along this stretch you'll see camellias, cherry trees, and a profusion of daffodils.

At the bottom of Beechwood Drive, near its intersection with Overbrook Road, cross at the crosswalk and proceed along the gravel path, which begins across another bridge over Shades Creek. In a pleasant contrast to the manicured lawns you've just passed, nature's landscaping takes over here.

In early spring, on that first stretch of trail, wildflowers appear in abundance: trillium, spring beauty, rue anemone, bluets against the moss-covered roots of an oak. No matter the season, the beech trees have their appeal, standing straight and tall beside the running waters.

The gravel nature trail continues 0.6 mile until it intersects Overbrook Road. Carefully cross Overbrook at the crosswalk.

Here begins Jemison Trail. It is paved and winds through the woods, by the creek and out to the roadside, through Jemison Park. Along the way there are benches, picnic tables, and spur trails. The only tricky part is on this eastern end, where a series of elevated concrete steps takes you across Shades Creek. They're easy to navigate under normal conditions, but after a heavy rain they're submerged and impassable.

Jemison Park is named for Robert Jemison, Mountain Brook's founder and visionary. Jemison was one of the great optimistic voices for Birmingham and led several development efforts, urban and suburban, residential and commercial, including Roebuck Springs, portions of Forest Park, the city of Fairfield, and of course, his crowning project, Mountain Brook.

Mountain Brook was built with a reverent attitude toward the natural landscape that was rooted in the ideas championed by Frederick Law Olmsted, the designer of Central Park. This parkway is a good place to think about how Jemison and his planners left natural areas not only for the sake of beauty but also out of the practical recognition that floodplains flood.

The original vision of Mountain Brook is still being realized. The development was still in its infancy when the stock market crashed in 1929. As late as the 1970s, the Jemison Park area was a flood-prone, privet-chocked thicket. Only in the past couple of decades has the park been cleared and cared for. The well-used and well-loved trail system in the park is just one part of a widespread network of sidewalks and trails the city has built in recent years. It's an investment in the life and health of the community.

Aside from the natural attractions of this hike, the grand homes on the opposite side of Mountain Brook Parkway, with their various architectural styles, command attention.

In particular, you'll notice one white-columned mansion on the Shades Creek side of Mountain Brook Parkway. This was a model house for the original Jemison development and was built to resemble George Washington's ancestral home, Mount Vernon. If you've ever seen the movie *Stay Hungry,* you'll recognize this house. Filmed in Birmingham in the 1970s, *Stay Hungry* featured Arnold Schwarzenegger's first speaking role and costarred Jeff Bridges and Sally Field.

Opposite the model home is the Old Mill, also part of Jemison's original development and the iconic landmark of Mountain Brook. This mill was built on the site of Perryman's Mill, a gristmill that operated from 1867 to 1887. The replica mill functioned as a teahouse and attraction for potential homebuyers. It later became (and still is) a private residence.

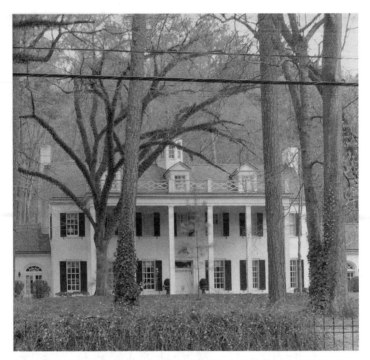

BUILT TO RESEMBLE MOUNT VERNON, THIS HOME ON MOUNTAIN BROOK PARKWAY WAS THE CENTERPIECE OF THE ORIGINAL DEVELOPMENT.

Jemison Trail ends just short of Mountain Brook Parkway's intersection with Cahaba Road. Here you can see more of the stone entrance gates that mark the boundaries of the original Jemison development.

Crossing Mountain Brook Parkway, follow the Watkins Trace Trail, a gravel path along Watkins Creek, a feeder creek to Shades Creek.

The creekside trail wanders a secluded ravine until it emerges to cross Watkins Road. On the other side, it becomes a paved walkway alongside Cahaba Road.

Now you're back at the edge of Mountain Brook Village. Find some refreshment or find your car. Before you leave, take a look around.

There has been a lot of attention paid over the years to maintaining the scale and architectural consistency of the village, and some major additions and renovations are under way. The initial plans sparked controversy and conversation about whether, with the new development, the village would preserve the character established by the founders. See what you think.

Nearby Attractions

The **Birmingham Zoo** (2630 Cahaba Rd.; 205-879-0409, **birminghamzoo .com**) and **Birmingham Botanical Gardens** (2612 Lane Park Rd.; 205-414-3950, **bbgardens.org**) are both just outside of Mountain Brook Village. The village itself has a wide array of eating, drinking, and shopping options.

Directions

From Mountain Brook Village, head east on Montevallo Road. The oldest house in Shades Valley will be on your right after 2.8 miles. Just beyond that, about 3 miles from Mountain Brook Village, at the intersection of Euclid Avenue and Montevallo Road, take a right onto Leach Drive. After passing one street on your left, bear left onto Groover Drive. After crossing Shades Creek, Groover becomes Shiloh Drive. Reach a stop sign. Turn right onto Stone River Road and go up the hill. Stay on Stone River, looking for a blue historical marker on your right. Across the street from the marker is a gravel parking area. For exploring individual segments, there are several parking areas along the route, including one at Overbrook Road and Beechwood Drive, another at Overbrook and Park Brook Road (a short extension of Overbrook near the intersection with Mountain Brook Parkway), and several gravel lots along Mountain Brook Parkway.

7

Shades Creek Greenway & Homewood Forest Preserve

SCENERY: ★ ★ ★
TRAIL CONDITION: ★ ★
CHILDREN: ★ ★ ★
DIFFICULTY: ★ ★ ★
SOLITUDE: ★ ★ ★ ★ ★

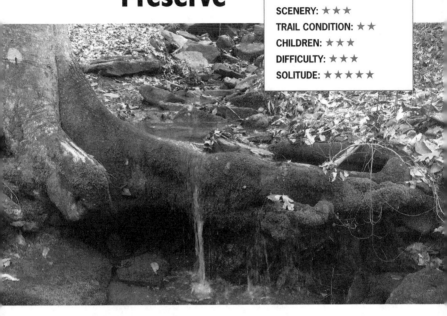

GPS TRAILHEAD COORDINATES: N33° 27.615' W86° 47.482'

DISTANCE & CONFIGURATION: 2.6-mile loop (with several alternatives described on the opposite page, ranging from 1 to 5 miles)

HIKING TIME: 1.5 hours

HIGHLIGHTS: Shades Creek and Shades Mountain, spring wildflowers and fall color, paved and bustling greenway, solitary mountainside hike with views of Shades Valley

ELEVATION: 625' at Homewood Forest Preserve Trailhead, 632' at suggested trailhead (University Park Place), 765' at peak

ACCESS: No restrictions or admission, but some options will require a little thought when you're finding a place to park.

MAPS: Available at the website below

FACILITIES: None

WHEELCHAIR ACCESS: Shades Creek Greenway is paved and wheelchair-accessible; Homewood Forest Preserve is not.

COMMENTS: Homewood Forest Preserve trail can get overgrown in late summer.

CONTACT: Shades Creek Greenway, **trekbirmingham.com/places/shades-creek-greenway**; Homewood Forest Preserve, **shadescreek.org**

Overview

This hike combines the virtues of two venues: Shades Creek Greenway and Homewood Forest Preserve. The greenway is a paved trail along Lakeshore Drive that makes a great place to walk, run, or ride a bike, without interaction with automobiles. It features Shades Creek and some nice floodplain forest. Homewood Forest Preserve offers a moderately vigorous mountain climb into an intact forest, a close encounter with a pocket of wilderness in the midst of urban development.

Route Details

I'm going to describe a 3-mile loop that combines a portion of the Shades Creek Greenway, starting near the campus of Samford University, with the Homewood Forest Preserve. Before I launch into that, I want to mention other options that can provide variety or additional distance. You can park at the greenway's western trailhead off South Lakeshore Drive near the Homewood soccer fields and make this into a 5-mile loop. You can park at the eastern trailhead at Brookwood Village and make a 3-mile balloon loop. Or you can park on the east side of Homewood High School in the high school's parking lot and hike only the Homewood Forest Preserve loop (about 1 mile by itself).

I'm going to split the difference and recommend parking on the street on University Park Place, off Lakeshore Drive near Homewood High School. University Park Place can be accessed by the bridge crossing Shades Creek, opposite the west entrance gate to Samford University.

To access the trail, look for a metal guardrail on the Homewood High School side of the bridge over Shades Creek. A footpath cuts through here to the trail and its pedestrian bridge across Shades Creek.

The hike I'm proposing heads upstream, to the east from here, but I'll note that the stretch of greenway heading west and ending at the Homewood Soccer Complex has much to offer. It passes through a floodplain forest that has grown out of what was once a 117-acre lake, Edgewood Lake. Development of the lake began in 1913. It was

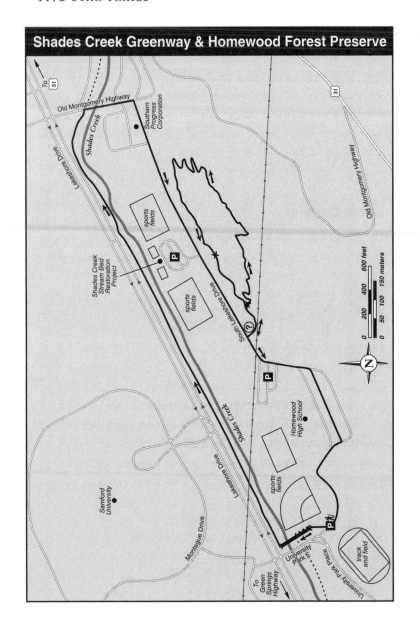

Shades Creek Greenway & Homewood Forest Preserve

formed by damming Shades Creek. Reachable by a streetcar that ran down Homewood's Broadway Street, it was a popular recreation and picnic spot. There were grand plans to create a motor speedway around the lake, patterned after the one in Indianapolis. The north and south runs eventually became Lakeshore and South Lakeshore Drives, but the raceway was never completed. The dam broke on several occasions, and the lake was drained in 1946.

From its bed grew a forest of beech trees, tulip poplars, sycamores, and oaks, mixed with an understory clogged with privet and other invasive plants. Completed in 1999, the Shades Creek Greenway cut through this tangle, though the work of battling the invasive privet continues. Winding side trails have been developed along this stretch, creating more mileage for walking and riding.

Our walk, however, heads east, upstream, with Samford University across the street on the left. As you progress, enjoy the river birches and redbud trees planted along the trail, as well as the view of the university campus. Samford's roots go back to 1842, but this campus opened in 1957. Immaculately landscaped and perched on the hillside, it looks older, with its stately live oaks and redbrick Georgian Colonial–style architecture. The school has a total enrollment of more than 4,600 students in the undergraduate college and graduate programs in law, business, education, and health sciences.

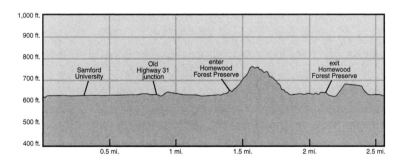

After passing the Samford main gate, turn your attention back to the greenway and the creek. As with most of our urban waterways, Shades Creek has its natural beauty but also bears the bruises of flowing through the human landscape. When it rains, the creek swells rapidly. Some of that is natural, of course, but its volume and velocity are increased as a side effect of development upstream. Rainwater surges into the creek, channeled there by the storm sewers that gather runoff from roads and parking lots. With the surge comes trash. You'll often see discarded plastic shopping bags dangling from tree limbs and all sorts of other debris, from plastic bottles to basketballs, floating downstream or stranded on the banks.

Despite those blemishes, the creek retains a natural beauty. Herons wade in the shallows, fishing for minnows. Water tumbles over rocks and drops. In this stretch, some of those water features are a man-made attempt to help the creek heal itself.

Consulting with hydrologists and biologists, Samford University installed a series of cross vanes in the creek—V-shaped configurations of large boulders spanning the width of the stream. The upstream point of the cross vane causes water to slow down along the bank and speed up in the center of the stream. This decreases stream-bank erosion, allows sediment to drop out of the water, and creates pools and pockets of habitat for aquatic wildlife. It seems to be working. Every once in a while, I see a fly-fisherman wading in the creek and casting in this area.

Continue on the greenway to its intersection with Old Montgomery Highway. Take a right on the road. Watch for traffic as you cross the bridge and walk up toward the intersection with South Lakeshore Drive, where you'll turn right and head toward Homewood High School.

This stretch of road hosts an unusual wildlife event: the annual running of the spotted salamanders. After the first warm rain of the year, the salamanders, dark in color with bright-yellow spots, emerge from their lairs on Shades Mountain and scramble across the road, headed for pools of water on the Shades Creek side of the road. There they perform a courtship dance and do a little lovemaking. Volunteers monitor the weather and try to catch the migration so they can protect the amphibians from passing traffic.

Near the parking lot for Homewood High School, a power-line right-of-way descends Shades Mountain. The Homewood Forest Preserve trailhead and a kiosk are located on the right-of-way. After the kiosk, the trail turns left into the woods, passes through a wetland, and crosses a bridge.

I work on the Samford campus and sometimes walk at lunch to escape from the computer screen. I enjoy the walk on the greenway, but it's in this first little stretch that my mind begins to clear and I start focusing on what's at my feet. One of my favorite things about this book project was taking a series of hikes at the forest preserve from March through April, watching spring come little by little, day by day.

First, the trilliums popped up out of subterranean hiding. Then came other wildflowers: rue-anemone, tiny bluets, and bloodroot. They changed daily, pushing to bloom before the tree canopy returned and shaded out these spring ephemerals. I watched the trillium spread its green spotted leaves, then push up from the center a green protrusion that would become its bloom. Over the course of days, the trillium subtly opened to reveal its maroon petals. It gave me an extra reason to get up in the morning to see what came next. There seemed a message in this ancient ritual, a reminder to seize the day.

The second phase of my decompression happens at the trickling stream you walk beside as you head up the mountain. In wet weather, a drainage descending the mountain here drops down from a shelf formed by the muscular roots of beech trees. That creates the soothing sight and sound of a miniature waterfall.

Pass an outdoor classroom on your right and continue up the hill, noticing the wide variety of trees: shagbark hickory, magnolia, and beech, along with loblolly, longleaf, and Virginia pines. On a recent hike, I came eye-to-eye with a barred owl that was perched on a low branch not far off the trail. I stayed still, and we stared at each other for several moments. He decided I wasn't a threat, turned his attention back down the hillside, and shortly swooped away in pursuit of prey.

As you continue climbing the ridge, avoid the spur trails that shoot off toward the right-of-way and more directly up the mountain. The trail peaks and evens out around 765 feet in elevation (you started at 632 feet just a quarter-mile ago). As you walk along at this elevation, look back to the west and you can see the Samford library and the tops of other campus buildings, as well as buildings on the campus of Southern Progress, the division of Time Inc. that publishes *Southern Living* and other magazines. At the far eastern edge of the forest preserve, above Covenant Presbyterian Church, you can look out over the valley and see Brookwood Village shopping and office complex and the surrounding hillsides.

As you begin your descent along a series of switchbacks, you'll be surrounded by juvenile maple trees, which light up red when the leaves change. It's a great spot for a fall leaf pilgrimage.

Your return along the base of the mountain, paralleling South Lakeshore, is a nice spot for wildflowers as well. When you follow the path back off the power-line right-of-way and reach the road, turn left toward Homewood High School.

You'll have to hike up Shades Mountain again, this time following South Lakeshore through the high school's parking area.

Descend on the other side of the high school and continue heading west on South Lakeshore until you reach the intersection with University Park Place, where the hike began. Unfortunately, there are no sidewalks along this stretch, so use caution.

Nearby Attractions

Samford University welcomes visitors. Information and maps are available at The Hub, at the University Center. Call 205-726-2407.

Brookwood Village, where the Shades Creek Greenway originates in the east, offers a wide variety of restaurants and shops.

Directions

Suggested trailhead: To access the trail near Samford University, turn off Lakeshore Drive onto University Park East, which becomes University Park Place, opposite the west gate (not the main gate) of Samford University. That turn is 2.7 miles east of I-65 (at Exit 255) and 1.8 miles west of US 280. Cross the creek and take a right to find street parking along University Park Place.

Western trailhead: From the intersection of Green Springs Highway and Lakeshore Drive, go south on Green Springs (signed as Columbiana Road farther south) and take the first left onto South Lakeshore Drive; then take the first left into the trailhead parking lot. If you're coming north on Columbiana Road, it's the last right turn before the Green Springs–Lakeshore intersection.

Eastern trailhead: At the corner of Brookwood Boulevard and Brookwood Village Road in Homewood. Park near the Target store at Brookwood Village.

8

Vestavia Hills
Library in the Forest

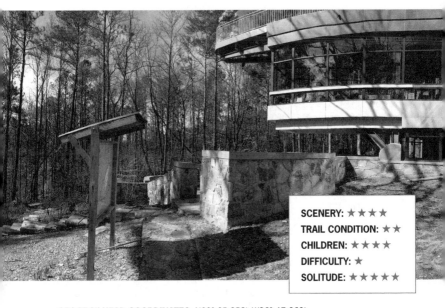

> **SCENERY:** ★ ★ ★ ★
> **TRAIL CONDITION:** ★ ★
> **CHILDREN:** ★ ★ ★ ★
> **DIFFICULTY:** ★
> **SOLITUDE:** ★ ★ ★ ★ ★

GPS TRAILHEAD COORDINATES: N33° 25.858' W86° 47.260'

DISTANCE & CONFIGURATION: 0.9-mile loop

HIKING TIME: 1 hour

HIGHLIGHTS: Small stream bordered by beech trees, some quite large. Larger boulders downstream and a waterfall at the far end of the route. Mixed pine–hardwood forest on the ridge of the canyon opposite the library.

ELEVATION: 680' at library trailhead, 560' at Vestavia Hills Elementary Central trailhead

ACCESS: Library hours: Monday–Thursday, 9 a.m.–8 p.m.; Friday–Saturday, 9 a.m.–6 p.m.; and Sunday, 1–5 p.m. When the library is closed, the trail can be accessed by walking around the library on the side closest to US 31 (to the right when facing the front entrance).

MAPS: On the kiosk at the library trailhead; another map of the trail system is posted at the Vestavia Hills Elementary Central trailhead.

FACILITIES: Beyond the offerings you expect of a library—books, computers, videos, restrooms, and air-conditioning—the Library in the Forest has some of the most pleasant places to read or work you'll find anywhere, both inside and outside.

WHEELCHAIR ACCESS: The library is wheelchair-accessible; the Boulder Canyon Trail is not.

COMMENTS: Bring a bag to pick up trash that inevitably washes into the canyon. Also, you might run into some treacherous conditions at creek crossings during and after heavy rains.

CONTACT: 205-978-0155, **vestavialibrary.org**

Overview

This hike is unique in that its central attraction is a building: Vestavia Hills Library in the Forest. It's a masterpiece. But yes, there is a hike here. It follows a headwater stream of Patton Creek as it drops through Boulder Canyon. Downstream from the library, near Vestavia Hills Elementary School Central, a waterfall is hidden away. You'll find a few longleaf pines on the ridges and some grand beech trees along the creek, which is pretty but shows the strains of draining its urbanized surroundings—it's hard to ignore the trash and erosion.

Route Details

If you haven't visited the Library in the Forest in Vestavia Hills, go.

Opened in 2010, the 35,000-square-foot library is styled with a mix of the region's traditional sandstone and angular modern design. It was the state's first LEED (Leadership in Energy and Environmental Design)–certified library and includes such eco-friendly features as a rooftop garden, a rainwater collection and storage system, and low-energy lighting. Perched on the hillside that drops off to the creek and canyon, the library feels integrated into the surrounding woods. Towering glass walls in the rear of the building create the feeling that you're in a tree house (albeit one with climate control). It's an ideal place to hang out and read or work, and when you've grown tired of sitting, right out the back door are a creek and a trail to explore.

To reach the trail from within the library, descend to the bottom floor and look for stairs and a door leading out the rear. Once outside, head downhill and pick up the stone path and stairs. At the edge of the forest are two circular patios partially enclosed by low stone walls. Both have large boulders in the center.

Have a seat if you like, or continue descending the stone stairs, bordered by mountain laurel, into the canyon.

A bridge crosses the creek here, and the surrounding area is idyllic. Small waterfalls punctuate the creek. In the summer there is

Vestavia Hills Library in the Forest

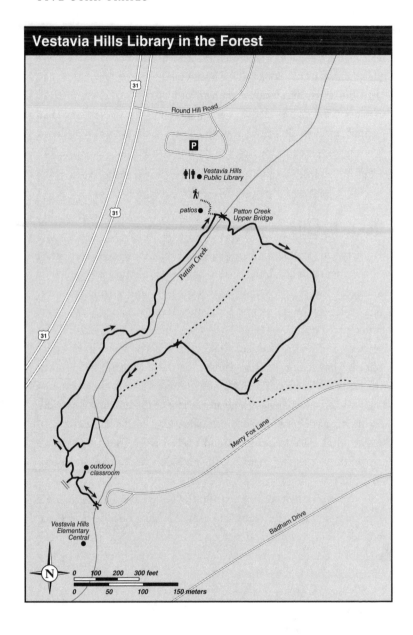

Round Hill Road

31

P

Vestavia Hills
Public Library

patios●

Patton Creek
Upper Bridge

Patton Creek

31

31

Merry Fox Lane

● outdoor
classroom

Vestavia Hills
Elementary
Central
●

Badham Drive

N

| 0 | 100 | 200 | 300 feet |

| 0 | 50 | 100 | 150 meters |

deep shade, and in the winter you'll enjoy the beech trees with their crinkled copper leaves.

You can pursue a loop here in either direction, with a few side options along the way.

I crossed the bridge and hiked up the hill on the opposite bank. Along the way, signs identify the variety of tree species on the mountainside. You'll note a trail diverging to the right (southwest)—you can take this for a slightly shorter walk or continue uphill to the path that follows the top and back sides of the little ridge forming the canyon. Both are nice, and they reconnect a little farther down the line. Up on the ridge, you are aware that you're not deep in the woods. Dogs bark from suburban backyards. The traffic on US 31 is audible. But you've at least halfway escaped. And outside of the area close to the library, I never encountered anyone else on the trail.

Once the high road and the low road have reconnected, you'll descend to the creek and cross it. This is a fun little crossing, with easy transit under normal conditions across very large boulders.

On the opposite side of the creek, continue following the creek downstream along the trail. This area is slightly confusing to navigate because you'll encounter some offshoot trails. You'll be fine if you keep going downstream, passing an outdoor classroom on the way to the final bridge and the Vestavia Hills Elementary Central trailhead.

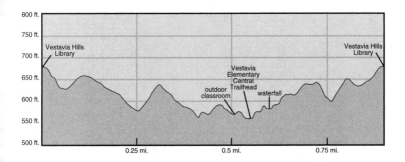

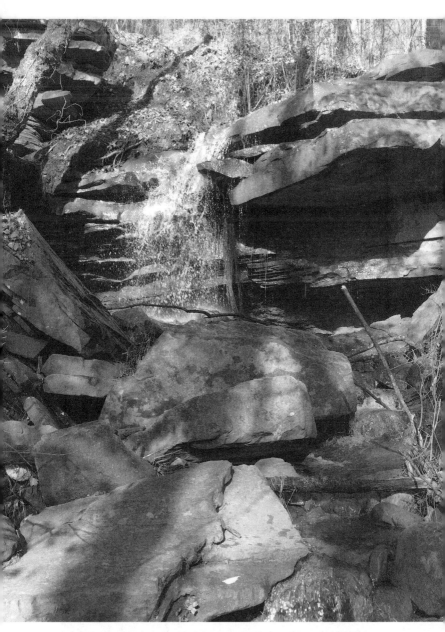

A WATERFALL IN BOULDER CANYON, DOWNSTREAM FROM THE LIBRARY

From here you'll start off by retracing your steps, but stay left, looking for a path that takes you up to a branch of the creek that comes down from the US 31 edge of the canyon. Hidden up that branch is a decent-sized waterfall.

After taking in the sights there, head back on that side of the canyon. A spur trail leads up to US 31, but you don't need to check it out. You'll also encounter a spur that leads back down to the main stem of the creek where you previously crossed. Stay on the side of the creek (the left side if you're facing upstream) and follow the path back up toward the library. This portion of the route stays uphill from the creek, then drifts down and runs alongside it up to the bridge.

Nearby Attractions

On your way to or from the library, check out the **Sibyl Temple,** high atop Shades Mountain off US 31 South, just as you enter Vestavia Hills from the north. The circular, white-columned building is a replica of the Temple of Sibyl in Tivoli, Italy. The temple once served as the gazebo entrance to the gardens of the estate of George Ward, a mayor of Birmingham in the early 20th century. Ward's home, which he named Vestavia, was designed in the style of the Roman Temple of Vesta and stood where Vestavia Hills Baptist Church stands today. The landmark offers sweeping views of Shades Valley.

Directions

The Vestavia Hills Library in the Forest is located at 1221 Montgomery Highway, just off US 31 and south of the main entrance to the Vestavia Hills Civic Center. Access to the library parking lot is off Round Hill Road, on the opposite side of the highway from the civic center and sports fields (the eastern side). Coming from I-65, take Exit 252 and head north on US 31.

Moss Rock Preserve (Hikes 9–11)

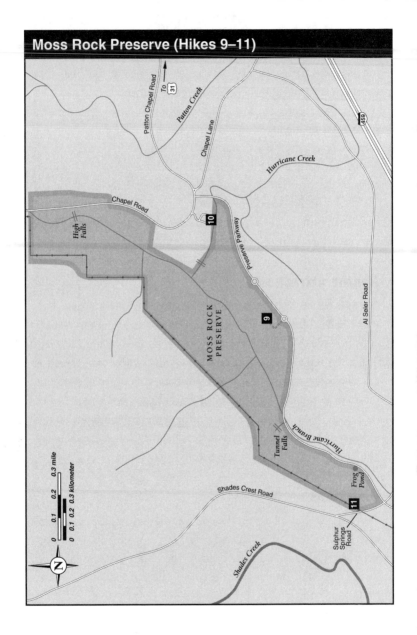

Moss Rock Preserve

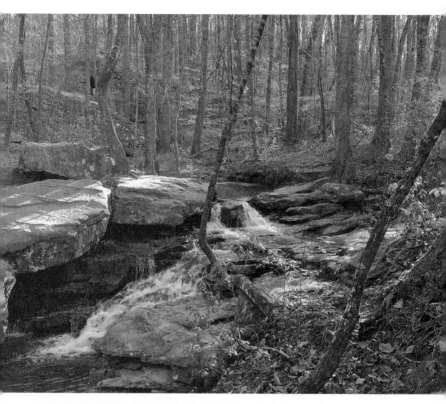

HURRICANE BRANCH SNAKES ITS WAY THROUGH THE PRESERVE.

Moss Rock Preserve Overview

MOSS ROCK PRESERVE IS SOMETHING OF A MIRACLE. Right in the middle of Hoover's suburban boom is this 350-acre wooded oasis that features waterfalls, biologically and geologically rare sandstone glades, challenging hills, great views, and, most famously, an assemblage of giant boulders that makes it a regional attraction for rock climbers. Throughout the park, along 12 miles of well-marked trails, you'll find rock formations to explore, wildflowers to see, and well-made signage that identifies plant species.

Moss Rock Preserve was made possible by persistent advocacy from citizens, forward-thinking action by the city of Hoover, and cooperation with U.S. Steel, which owned the land and is developing the adjacent housing community, The Preserve. It's been lovingly cared for and developed by the Friends of Moss Rock Preserve, local Boy Scout troops, neighbors, and volunteers.

The city began acquiring the land for the park in 1992 and dedicated the initial 250 acres as a park in 2000. Later acquisitions in 2007 and 2008 made for the 100-acre expansion, Boulder Gorge, which was dedicated in 2012.

Because Moss Rock is really cool, really close to civilization, and relatively compact, it gets a lot of use. With the continued development of The Preserve (the housing community), that use will likely continue to grow.

It's incumbent on all of us to take care of Moss Rock. Unfortunately, you see plenty of evidence (in the form of fire rings and trash) that some people are abusing this asset. If you visit, bring a trash bag and fight back against litter.

Every visit to Moss Rock has provided me with surprises. I had visited the Boulder Field, which is a great place for kids of all ages to explore. I knew there was a creek around there, but I didn't know how pretty Hurricane Branch was when the water is really flowing. Nor had I seen the numerous waterfalls that, in wet weather, tumble down Shades Mountain on the way to the creek. I was particularly blown away by the 30-foot tumble of High Falls, the crown jewel of the newest addition to Moss Rock, Boulder Gorge. I was also "shocked" by the scenic highlights and rugged challenge of the Powerline Trail.

Moss Rock Preserve centers on two branches of Hurricane Creek running along a narrow valley between the slope of Shades Mountain to the north and Pine Mountain to the south. Those two branches converge and flow out of the park by Simmons Middle School.

Trailheads

You can access Moss Rock from three trailheads, each with its own virtues:

SIMMONS MIDDLE SCHOOL LOWER PARKING LOT 1575 Patton Chapel Rd. Coming from US 31, this is just past the intersection with Preserve Parkway. This trailhead primarily serves the Boulder Gorge (Orange) Trail, with connections to the rest of the system.

BOULDER FIELD PARKING LOT 617 Preserve Parkway, adjacent to the commercial center at The Preserve. Provides access to the White Trail, Hurricane Branch, the sandstone glade, and Boulder Field (large sandstone formations that draw visitors from around the region).

SULPHUR SPRINGS PARKING LOT Gravel lot on Sulphur Springs Road, between Shades Crest Road and Preserve Parkway. When parking at this lot, please don't block the Alabama Power Company service gate.

Trails

The **Red, White,** and **Blue Trails** serve the southwestern two-thirds of the preserve, including Hurricane Branch, Boulder Field, and the slopes of Shades Valley. The **Orange Trail** loops through the northeastern third, known as Boulder Gorge. The **Powerline Trail** traces the northern perimeter of both, along the power-line right-of-way.

RED TRAIL Leaves from Patriotic Junction, crosses Preserve Parkway, and winds through the woods on the opposite side of the street.

It's a pleasant walk, but, at least in winter, you can see the backs of houses that front a street at the top of the ridge. The trail crosses back over the parkway and reconnects to the White Trail.

WHITE TRAIL Starts at Patriotic Junction and travels to the Simmons Middle School parking lot, spending much of its course along Hurricane Branch. This is the low side of the property, though the White does offer a spur on its northeastern end that climbs the slope to Turtle Rock and Window Rock, offering connections to the Blue Trail and the Powerline Trail. Along the creek, the trail is easy and flat; in the northeast, the elevation gain presents more of a challenge.

BLUE TRAIL Traverses the forest of the upper mountainside, including some patches of longleaf pine. Some of the more remote boulders, such as the Great Wall, lie along the Blue. Spurs that climb the slopes are also generally blazed blue. One particularly scenic spur runs between Hurricane Creek and the main Blue Trail, climbing along a creek that tumbles down a rocky course on the southwestern edge of the Sandstone Glade. The Blue has some elevation gain and loss, requiring moderate exertion.

ORANGE TRAIL Accessible from the White Trail, the Orange Trail is a loop that begins at the confluence of two branches of Hurricane Branch. The Orange follows a branch upstream, to the northeast and toward the surprising and impressive High Falls. The path along the southeastern bank of the creek, closest to Chapel Road, is an easy streamside walk. The trail spur up to the Top of the World Boulders (across Chapel Road) is steep but rewarding. The Orange loop on the opposite bank climbs the slope, then descends back to the creek at Rock House Boulders.

POWERLINE TRAIL Running from the Sulphur Springs parking lot to the far northwest corner of the park, this rugged trek along the power-line right-of-way is surprisingly beautiful. Because it is cleared of trees, sunlight pours in, producing an abundance of wildflowers of the type you don't see in the forest. The open sky offers some arresting views of the surrounding countryside. As in the rest of the park, you'll find unusual rock formations, from large boulders to Moon Rock, another sandstone-glade ecosystem.

Suggested loops are described on the following pages. For a truly epic loop, start at the Sulphur Springs parking lot, take the White Trail past Boulder Field, and connect to the Orange Trail. Hike the length of Boulder Gorge, past High Falls and up to Top of the World. Return across Chapel Road and follow the service road out to its connection with the Powerline Trail for a grueling but scenic return along rough terrain. It adds up to about 6 miles, and with so much up and down, you end up with a total ascent of more than 1,000 feet over the course of the hike.

More Information

DIRECTIONS: Moss Rock Preserve can be accessed from US 31 via Patton Chapel Road or from Sulphur Springs Road, off Shades Crest Road in Bluff Park. The main entrance within the Preserve neighborhood is on Preserve Parkway.

ACCESS: Sunrise–sunset; no charge

MAPS: An excellent trail map is available at the Hoover city website, **hooveral.org.** Click on the "Visitors" tab and follow the link to Moss Rock Preserve; then follow the link to "Map and Trail Guide." For the best map version, click on "Color Trail Map Produced for Moss Rock." Also available are informative species lists and a trail guide. **Trek Birmingham (trekbirmingham .com)** also has a nice description of the geology and ecology of the area.

FACILITIES: Excellent signage and well-maintained trails, but no developed facilities. At the preserve trailhead, there's a restaurant called **The Boot at Preserve Village** (616 Preserve Pkwy.; 205-978-8988, **thebootatpreservevillage.vpweb.com**). Its hours are a little unusual; it closes between 2 p.m. and 4 p.m., and it's open only from 11 a.m. to 2 p.m. on Sundays. Closed Mondays.

WHEELCHAIR ACCESS: None

COMMENTS: Dogs are welcome but must be leashed.

CONTACT: City of Hoover, **hooveral.org/?nid=214**

Moss Rock Preserve:
Boulder Field

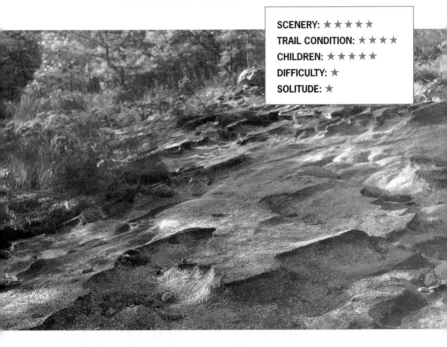

SCENERY: ★ ★ ★ ★ ★
TRAIL CONDITION: ★ ★ ★ ★
CHILDREN: ★ ★ ★ ★ ★
DIFFICULTY: ★
SOLITUDE: ★

GPS TRAILHEAD COORDINATES: N33° 22.899' W86° 50.415'

DISTANCE & CONFIGURATION: Well under a mile out-and-back to the Boulder Field, with options for miles and miles beyond that. If you're up for an out-and-back of close to 2 miles or a loop of 2.5 miles, throw in a jaunt to Turtle Rock, a unique boulder on the mountainside with a nice view. That expedition can be made into a loop using the Blue Trail.

HIKING TIME: Anywhere from no time to hours

HIGHLIGHTS: A collection of huge sandstone boulders form a natural playground, drawing everyone from children to serious rock climbers. Clear, clean Hurricane Branch is fed by waterfall tributaries in wet weather. A sandstone outcropping across the creek creates an unusual landscape of lichens, moss, rare flowers, and stunted trees.

ELEVATION: Start at 680', descend to 553', and climb to a peak at Turtle Rock at 735'.

ACCESS, MAPS, FACILITIES: See previous page.

WHEELCHAIR ACCESS: No official access, but may be passable to Hurricane Branch in a wheelchair with off-road tires.

COMMENTS: Please take care of this place, particularly the sandstone glade, which is among only a handful of known examples of such a landscape in Alabama. Bring a trash bag and pack out what others have left behind.

Overview

The Shades Mountain Boulder Field at Moss Rock Preserve draws climbers from around the Southeast. From the trailhead off Preserve Parkway, it's a very short walk to see the weather-worn boulders, some 10–20 feet high, where boulderers climb challenging routes or "problems" across the face of the rock. At the base of the Boulder Field, Hurricane Branch carves its own path through rock formations, forming waterfalls along the way. Across the creek, you'll find a sandstone expanse with hardy but fragile plant communities specially adapted to the tough terrain. A well-marked nature trail along the creek offers options for further exploration.

Route Details

This is the classic introduction to Moss Rock Preserve, providing quick access to the park's top scenic and recreational highlights.

I'm listing the shortest possible distance to entice first-time hikers, but you can easily step it up with a trip to Turtle Rock (about 2 miles out-and-back from the parking lot, or in a loop that continues on the Blue Trail along the ridge before descending back along the edge of the sandstone glade).

Less than 100 yards from the parking lot, you enter a wonderland for rock climbing. In the early 1960s, John Gill, who is considered the father of modern bouldering, spent time climbing here and at other sites on Shades Mountain while working on his master's in mathematics at the University of Alabama. Now, 50 years later, you'll often see college kids headed out to free-climb on these rocks. Bouldering doesn't require much equipment: a foam crash pad for landing, maybe chalk, maybe shoes. But it does require upper- and lower-body strength, agility, grace, and know-how. It's fun to watch, and you'll discover some approachable climbs here.

Beyond bouldering, the rocks are just fun to explore. There are narrow crevices to navigate, cavelike openings to crawl through, and summits to reach. You could spend all day.

Moss Rock Preserve: Boulder Field

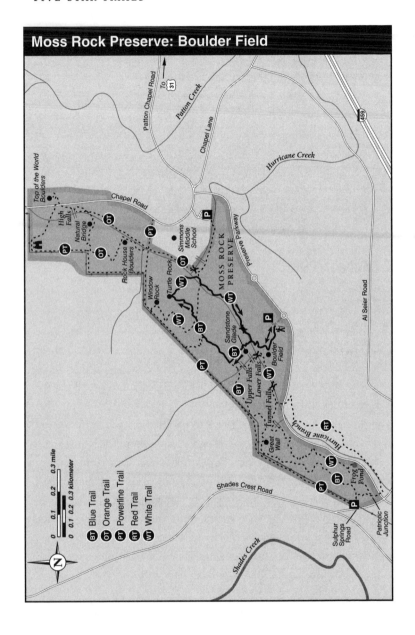

At the foot of the slope is Hurricane Branch. What's particularly nice about this section of the branch is that it's relatively free of trash and sediment pollution. That's because it originates close by and there isn't yet enough civilization to have damaged it too greatly. It has a sandy bottom in some stretches. In other stretches, it carves channels and chutes through a rocky course. The creek is shaded by mountain laurel and beech trees.

Crossing the creek and wandering a little in the downstream direction, you'll see a clearing just up the slope of Shades Mountain. Walk up to the edge and you'll see that the clearing is actually an expanse of exposed sandstone. The weathered surface at first looks barren, but on closer inspection you'll find it's covered with lichens and mosses. In small eroded pockets in the rock, there is enough soil to support hardy flowering plants, and in some of the deeper pockets are what look like young trees. These are actually old trees that have been growing very slowly, making careful use of the limited moisture and soil there. People do walk out on the sandstone and enjoy the open views and odd landscape of bonsai-like trees growing there. But tread lightly. As tough as this vegetation is, it can't take much human traffic.

On the southwestern side (to the left when you look up the slope) is a drainage that makes a great tumbling waterfall in the rainy season.

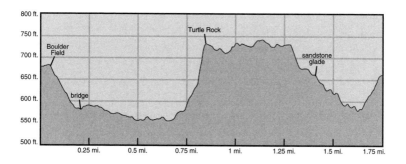

If you move downstream on the creek from the glade area along the White Trail, there's a well-marked Boy Scout–built nature trail that can help you get up to speed on your plant identification. You can also enjoy the drops and chutes of the water descending the branch.

If you want to make a little expedition of it, follow the White Trail down to and across a small dirt service road. You'll be offered the option of going right and back across the creek toward the Simmons Middle School Trailhead. Instead, stay straight and follow the White Trail as it ascends Shades Mountain. About 1 mile from the parking lot you reach Turtle Rock, a collection of humped boulders that, from the right angle, have the look of a giant sea turtle. If you mount the top of the turtle and peer out, you get a view of the valley and can spot the hotel tower at the Riverchase Galleria.

From here you can either retrace your route to the parking lot or proceed on the White Trail. If you choose to do the latter, you'll reach a junction that offers you the option of heading toward Window Rock. Instead, take the Blue Trail here, which continues at that elevation on the upper slope. You'll pass above the sandstone glade. Look carefully for a spur off the Blue Trail that heads downhill. That trail takes you back down to Hurricane Branch, and from there you can make your way back through Boulder Field to your car.

Directions

Park at the Boulder Field lot; see page 85 for details. See page 87 for general directions to the preserve.

Moss Rock Preserve:
Boulder Gorge Loop

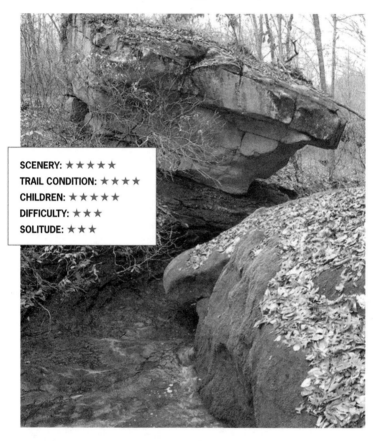

SCENERY: ★ ★ ★ ★ ★
TRAIL CONDITION: ★ ★ ★ ★
CHILDREN: ★ ★ ★ ★ ★
DIFFICULTY: ★ ★ ★
SOLITUDE: ★ ★ ★

GPS TRAILHEAD COORDINATES: N33° 23.143' W86° 49.940'

DISTANCE & CONFIGURATION: 3-mile loop (option for a 2-mile out-and-back)

HIKING TIME: 3 hours

HIGHLIGHTS: Multiple waterfalls, including High Falls, which tumbles about 30 feet down multiple cascades; the Top of the World Boulders, which offer a sweeping view of the surrounding country; and the Rock House Boulders, a series of "rooms" formed by nature

ELEVATION: 525' at low point, 793' at Top of the World Boulders

ACCESS, MAPS, FACILITIES, WHEELCHAIR ACCESS: See page 87.

COMMENTS: Please take care of this place. Bring a trash bag and pack out what others have left behind.

Moss Rock Preserve: Boulder Gorge Loop

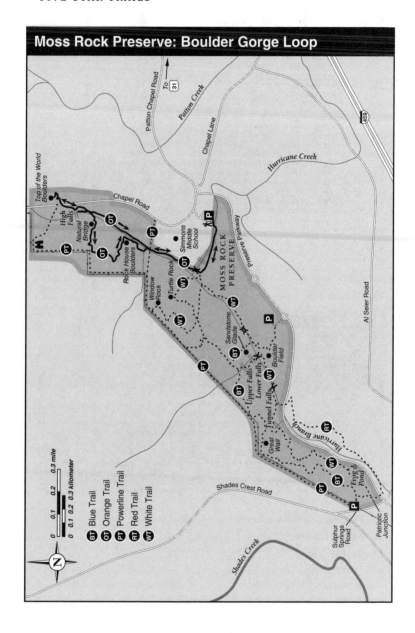

Patton Chapel Road

To 31

Patton Creek

Chapel Lane

Hurricane Creek

459

Top of the World Boulders

Chapel Road

High Falls

Natural Bridge

Rock House Boulders

Window Rock

Turtle Rock

Simmons Middle School

Preserve Parkway

M O S S   R O C K   P R E S E R V E

Sandstone Glade

Boulder Field

Upper Falls

Lower Falls

Tunnel Falls

Great Wall

Hurricane Branch

Al Seier Road

Frog Pond

Shades Crest Road

Patriotic Junction

Sulphur Springs Road

Shades Creek

0   0.1   0.2   0.3 mile
0   0.1   0.2   0.3 kilometer

BT Blue Trail
OT Orange Trail
PT Powerline Trail
RT Red Trail
WT White Trail

N

Overview

This loop starts with convenient parking at Simmons Middle School and follows Hurricane Branch upstream as it tumbles out the narrow valley between Pine Mountain and Shades Mountain. In wet weather, it offers multiple waterfalls as the stream winds through sandstone boulders. The climax comes at High Falls, a serious multi-stage waterfall. From there, a spur trail makes a steep uphill scramble to the Top of the World Boulders, which afford an expansive view of the valley. The return portion of the loop crosses the stream and climbs the Shades Mountain ridge a bit before descending to wind through the Rock House Boulders, a natural playground in sandstone with cavelike openings that invite hiding, climbing, and exploring.

Route Details

The Boulder Gorge Loop at Moss Rock Preserve covers the 99 acres that were formally added to Moss Rock in May 2012 by the city of Hoover, working in conjunction with the Freshwater Land Trust.

The city bought the property in 2007 for $4.55 million. A large apartment complex had been planned, and clearing for the project had begun. It's stunning to think what would have been lost if that project had proceeded.

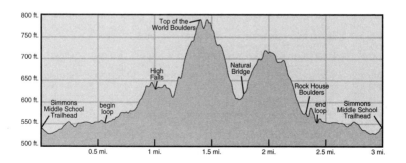

I was surprised at the pleasant walk up a lovely, boulder-strewn stream the first time I hiked the Boulder Gorge Loop. I was shocked when I reached High Falls, which must drop more than 30 feet over a series of falls. It would be an impressive destination deep in the woods, but this jewel is hidden just off Chapel Road.

Look for the information kiosk on the low side of the Simmons Middle School parking lot. There are sometimes trail maps here, but I'd recommend printing one at home (see page 87).

You begin by walking down a short hill from the parking lot to what appears to be an old road or sewer right-of-way. Take a right—the creek will be just ahead of you, and you'll be heading upstream. A short distance later, the white-blazed trail cuts left and crosses the stream over a series of rocks.

If the water is too high to cross, you can take the unmarked spur that you're already on; it will reconnect to the route farther down the trail. However, you should cross if you can. The stones are very stable, and on the other side you'll find a stand of mountain laurel and oakleaf hydrangea.

I could still make out Simmons Middle School by the time I reached the first set of small waterfalls. There had been rain in the two days prior, and the water volume was good. Even this simple waterfall was a relief. There's something about the sound of falling water that clears the storms in the synapses. I released a breath I didn't know I'd been holding through the tense traffic on I-65 and US 31.

At Trail Sign 9, a fork in the trail gives you a choice of going to Boulder Field and Turtle Rock or in the opposite direction to Boulder Gorge.

Go right (northeast) to Boulder Gorge, picking up the Orange Trail here and crossing back over Hurricane Branch. After crossing a bridge, you'll see sewer lines running along the creek—can't escape the fact that we live in an urbanized setting. The next stretch of trail is dense with privet. There is also mud and erosion from storm-sewer runoff.

You'll soon reach a fork in the trail; the loop you'll return on crosses the creek here. Continue straight, following the signs to High Falls. The scenery improves as you proceed.

Just after that junction you'll see a collection of huge boulders in the stream. If you have kids, you might want to turn them loose here and let them play in the creek and on the boulders. On the opposite bank, about halfway to High Falls, are the Rock House Boulders, which you'll thread your way through on the return loop.

In this collection of rock formations are cavelike openings and rooms to explore and hide out in. If you aren't intent on a hiking achievement, it would be a perfectly nice, short hike to frolic your way up the creek from here to High Falls and then call it a day.

To continue with the full agenda, continue upstream, enjoying the play of rocks and water and the native vegetation of the protected canyon.

At 0.8 mile, you reach a trail junction that you'll want to remember.

Here, you have four choices. One is to bear right up the hill and get a glancing view of High Falls on your way to Top of the World. The second is to follow the stream up to the base of High Falls and see the falls up close and beautiful. A third option is to turn around and go back the way you came. The fourth is to pivot and cross the creek just downstream of this intersection and follow the return side of the Orange loop.

For the purposes of this adventure, I'm recommending a direct assault on High Falls, then a side trip to Top of the World, and finally a return to this intersection to finish the loop.

High Falls was a revelation to me. You continue a short ways up the creek branch you've been following, and all of a sudden you're looking at a terraced stack of falls cut into an abrupt rise in the mountainside. You can carefully clamber up the rocks to get back into the almost-hidden upper ravine formed by the first set of falls. I can't believe I grew up in Birmingham and never knew it existed. High Falls rivals Oak Mountain's Peavine Falls.

And you're not done with surprises on this hike.

From High Falls, rejoin the Orange Trail and take the spur toward Top of the World. The trail takes you up to Chapel Road, then crosses the road on the way to the boulders. Once you're across the road, it's a little tricky to find where the trail heads up into the woods. The spur starts on Chapel Road, near the intersection with Verdure Lane.

Once you've found the trail, it's a short, steep climb to a glorious view from the boulders atop the ridge. Top of the World is another spot that made me shake my head and ask, *How did I not know of this place?*

As you make your return toward High Falls, you have another option for a diversion. Walk out on the gravel service road through the area that had been cleared for the apartment development. Near

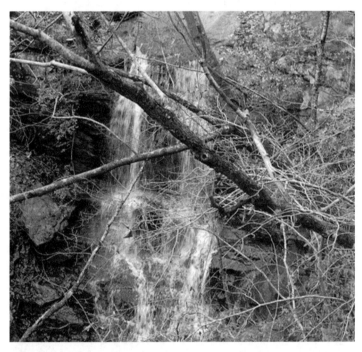

A HIGHLIGHT OF THE BOULDER GORGE LOOP, HIGH FALLS IS HIDDEN AWAY OFF CHAPEL ROAD.

the intersection with the Powerline Trail is another unexpected sweeping, scenic view.

Otherwise, retrace your steps to the intersection of trails near High Falls mentioned earlier. Cross the creek, following signs for a rock formation called Natural Bridge.

You can easily walk right past Natural Bridge. It's an interesting little formation that does look like a bridge, but it's quite petite.

Continuing past it, you ascend the mountainside, eventually encountering longleaf pine. Stands of longleaf are scattered throughout these ridges and would have been much more prevalent here when wildfires swept through on a regular basis. The Friends of Moss Rock have been doing what they can to clear the understory beneath longleaf stands to simulate the effect that fire would have on the landscape.

The trail is not particularly well marked in this area. Unofficial spurs and connections to other trails can lead you astray. To follow the official trail, you'll descend a drainage headed for the creek. This is leading you to the Rock House Boulders, which are on the opposite bank from the trail you hiked in on.

Rock House is certainly worth a visit. These rocks are smaller than the giant boulders of Boulder Field and have a natural-playground feel. Unfortunately, at least once when I visited, someone had built a campfire the night before and left trash strewn about and piled in a fire ring.

The Orange Trail continues along the hillside on that side of the creek until it intersects the power-line right-of-way. Turn left there, cross the creek, and follow the trail back out to the Simmons Middle School parking lot.

Directions

Park at the Simmons Middle School lower lot; see page 85 for details. See page 87 for general directions to the preserve.

Moss Rock Preserve:
Waterfall Loop from
Sulphur Springs Road

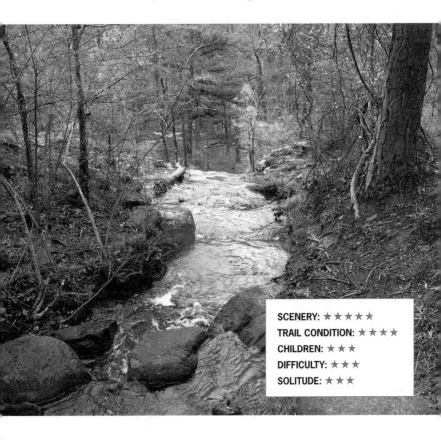

SCENERY: ★ ★ ★ ★ ★
TRAIL CONDITION: ★ ★ ★ ★
CHILDREN: ★ ★
DIFFICULTY: ★ ★ ★
SOLITUDE: ★ ★ ★

GPS TRAILHEAD COORDINATES: N33° 22.585' W86° 51.199'

DISTANCE & CONFIGURATION: 2.7-mile loop

HIKING TIME: 2 hours

HIGHLIGHTS: Waterfalls and wildflowers; boulders and sandstone glades; quiet and peace

ELEVATION: Start and end at 760', bottom out at 598', and climb to a peak of 790'.

ACCESS, MAPS, FACILITIES, WHEELCHAIR ACCESS: See page 87.

COMMENTS: Please take care of this place. Bring a trash bag and pack out what others
have left behind.

Overview

Leaving from the Sulphur Springs lot, this hike descends the slopes of Shades Mountain, picking up Hurricane Branch near its origins and following it into the center of Moss Rock Preserve at the Boulder Field. It then skirts the sandstone glade and climbs a spur of the Blue Trail up along a watercourse that has numerous waterfalls in wet weather. Connecting with the main Blue Trail, it winds through forest, past more remote rock formations, and makes its way back to the Sulphur Springs parking lot. Along the course of the hike, you hit the scenic highlights of the southwestern end of the preserve while enjoying more solitude than you'll find on the more heavily traveled routes in the park.

Route Details

I may have hit this hike on the best possible day of the year to enjoy its virtues. It was early April after healthy rains. The early-spring wildflowers were still out, and the dogwoods and redbuds had joined the chorus. Native azaleas had just burst onto the scene. Hurricane Branch was in full flow, and waterfalls cascaded down the edge of the sandstone glade, which was decorated with blooming yellow jasmine. It's enough of a route to get your blood pumping but short enough that you never feel like you're slogging.

I hope you're as lucky.

From the Sulphur Springs parking lot, you start on a spur of Blue Trail. When you meet the main Blue Trail, follow it downhill (right) to Patriotic Junction. On this early segment, informative signs identify the various tree species you're passing.

At Patriotic Junction, the Red, White, and Blue Trails meet. Get it?

Take the White Trail, headed toward Boulder Field, which is 1.3 miles from the junction. The White Trail is rather unremarkable at first. It's close to Preserve Parkway, and you can see the traffic. Early on, you're offered a side trail to Frog Pond, a wetland area right off Preserve Parkway. When I visited, it was too early to hear much

Moss Rock Preserve: Waterfall Loop from Sulphur Springs Road

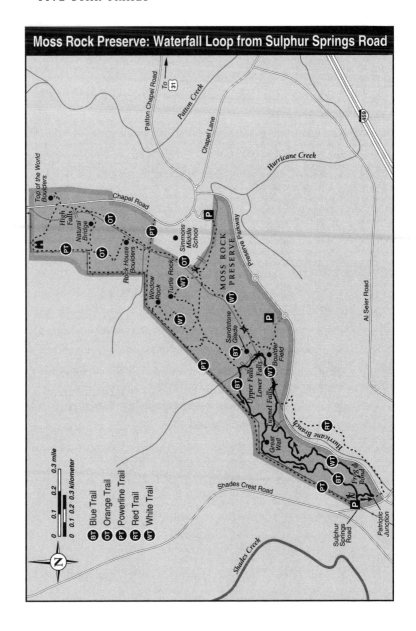

in the way of frog song. As you continue on the White Trail, it cuts back into the woods away from the Parkway and begins to get much more special: oakleaf hydrangea, red buckeye, dogwoods, and native azaleas appear. There were trillium and irises in bloom and even a few early coreopsis popping up.

You start encountering waterfalls at Tunnel Falls, which forms a natural bridge of sandstone across a mountain drainage. You continue to drop down to Hurricane Branch, which is as clear as pure spring water at this point in its journey. Along its course, large, moss-covered sandstone boulders start to appear.

The trail crosses the creek and reaches the famous Boulder Field. If you're taking a meandering walk, you can walk up and explore there.

When you're ready to proceed, look for another bridge crossing back to the opposite side of the creek, and find a trail sign that gives you a choice of going downstream (right) a few steps to the base of Lower Falls or proceeding up a Blue Trail spur toward the Upper Falls. Hopefully, the Lower Falls will be putting on a show for you, so check that out before you start your climb to the Upper Falls. Lower Falls spreads out over the western end of the large sandstone outcropping, which is visible up the slope to the right.

When you're ready to head up the Blue Trail toward the Upper Falls, take care not to be misled by the makeshift trails that lead back

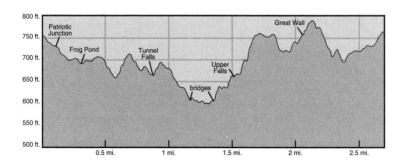

upstream. Once you do find the Blue and start climbing, you get a nice view of the edge of the sandstone glade. The hardy plants that make their homes here were putting on a show that afternoon, blooming yellow and blue against the rock that is accented with pale-green lichen.

As you climb, you parallel the tumbling watercourse. The trail crosses the drainage in the area of the Upper Falls. An open space sheltered by rocks here would make a nice place to pitch a tent if this were an overnight camping destination. It's not, but when I visited, it was apparent that some groups had gathered here the night before. Marring the otherwise-lovely scene were beer cans and plastic bottles floating in the pools. I gathered as many as I could fit in my pocket and was reminded again that I should always take along a trash bag.

Continue up the Blue spur until it meets the main Blue Trail. Here, take a left (to the west), following the trail signs toward Great Wall. There is one tricky spot along the way. The Blue sends a spur down the hill to meet the White and another up the hill headed for the Powerline Trail. Keep heading toward Great Wall, a grand but more isolated collection of large boulders. Enjoy scrambling up to the top if you want to feel like the king of the world. Follow the trail back out to the Sulphur Springs parking lot from here.

Directions

Park at the Sulphur Springs lot; see page 85 for details. See page 87 for general directions to the preserve.

A RAIN-FED CREEK TUMBLES DOWN SHADES MOUNTAIN ON THE WAY TO HURRICANE BRANCH.

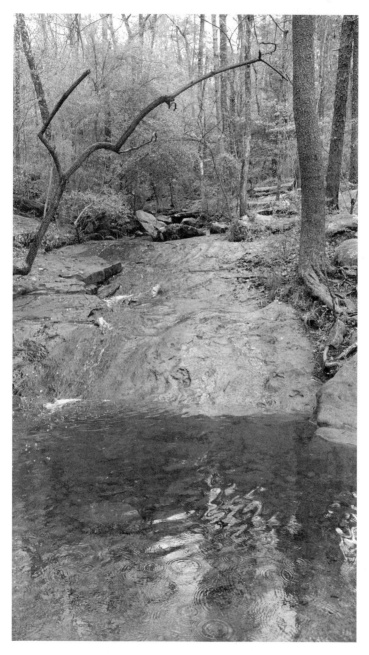

Oak Mountain State Park (Hikes 12–15)

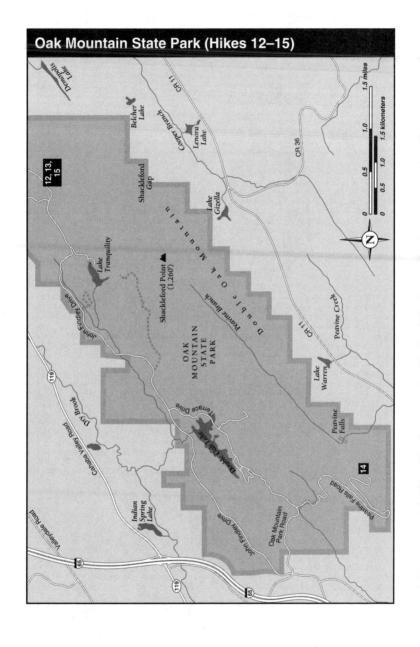

Oak Mountain
State Park

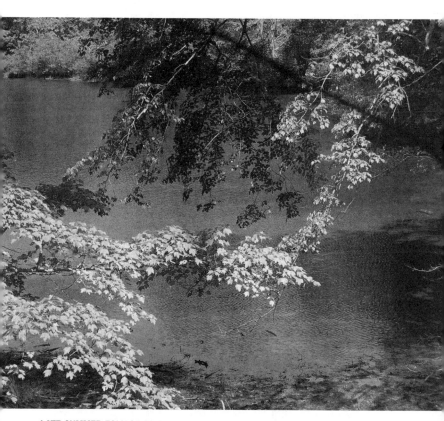

LATE-SUMMER FOLIAGE ON THE BANKS OF LAKE TRANQUILITY *(see Hike 13)*

Oak Mountain State Park Overview

AT 9,940 ACRES, Oak Mountain is Alabama's largest state park, smack-dab in the middle of the state's largest metro area. As long as you aren't trying to make the trek at rush hour, you can be on the trail to mountain overlooks or tumbling waterfalls in a matter of minutes, not hours.

Right in our backyard, we have 50 miles of trails on forested mountains and foothills, an extensive mountain-bike trail network, a BMX bicycle track, and a variety of other attractions, including three lakes, an interpretive center, a wildlife-rehabilitation center, a golf course, a demonstration farm, and horse stables. It's an easy day trip, or you could also choose a more extended stay by renting a cabin, staying in a developed or group campsite, or hiking to a backcountry campsite.

Despite all the activity, I've never felt crowded here. Sure, at peak seasons the trailhead parking lots tend to fill up, but once you're in the woods there's plenty of space.

You'll share some trails. You should be especially alert on Red Trails, which are open to use by mountain bikers. In fact, we should all be grateful to the mountain biking community, particularly Birmingham Urban Mountain Pedalers (BUMP), which maintains and in most cases built the Red Trail system. You might also cross paths with people riding horses, but most of the trails are reserved for hikers and runners. It takes just a little effort to get to stretches of trail you'll have largely to yourself.

My parents took me on my first hike at the park to Peavine Falls, a tradition that is alive and well today. As a family, we stayed at a cabin in the park, fished in the lake, and went on a trail ride. Later, when I was a Boy Scout, we took backpacking trips into the park's interior. We trained for the long-distance treks out west by hiking Oak Mountain's trails.

Over time, I became *too* familiar with Oak Mountain. So, after going away to school, moving back to Birmingham, and watching Hoover grow from a small crossroads suburb into a sprawling city, I stopped going south for my outdoor recreation.

But then, when I was asked to write this book, I went back. And I fell in love with the place all over again.

The park stretches about 8 miles along Double Oak Mountain. It's an appropriate name: Double Oak Mountain has two distinct ridges, or rims—a northern rim, which is roughly the path of the White Trail, and a southern rim, which is traced by the Blue Trail. In the center of the mountaintop is a forested valley. And along the north flank of the mountain is a succession of rising and falling draws and drainages—plenty of wooded real estate to explore.

The park was created through the State Land Act of 1927, initially at 940 acres. The National Park Service bought 8,000 acres to add to the park, and from 1934 to 1937, crews from the Depression-era Civilian Conservation Corps developed the initial roads, Lake Tranquility Dam, and pavilions and cabins.

Trailheads

The park's various trails come together in three places: the **North Trailhead,** in the northeast corner of the park, closest to the AL 119 entrance; the **South Trailhead,** at the southwestern end of Double Oak Lake, near the main entrance to the park; and the **Peavine Falls Parking Area,** at the end of Terrace Drive high atop Double Oak Mountain.

Trails

The hiking trails are color coded and well marked. Each is a little different in character and offers the hiker some variety. The **Red, White,** and **Blue Trails** all run from the low-elevation North Trailhead to high elevation at the Peavine Falls area.

RED TRAIL This is actually a system of trails. It includes the Red Road, the original dirt road through the park, stretching from the north trailhead to Ada Overlook near Peavine Falls. Because it is a road, it's wider than a typical hiking trail. You'll get nice views of Cahaba Valley at the trail's elevated southern end. At the north end, the trail runs alongside a stream that drains the mountaintop. The rest of the Red Trail system is a spiderweb of curvy trails on which hikers are allowed but which are primarily used by mountain bikers— an exception is the Red Trail around Double Oak Lake, which is enjoyed equally by hikers and bikers. Anywhere on the Red Trail, cyclists can sneak up on you fast, so be alert. Bikers coming up behind you will usually call ahead to apprise you of the fact. This *is* a mountain bike trail, after all, so just step aside and allow the rider to pass.

WHITE TRAIL This 6.4-mile-long trail runs a course similar to the Red, spending much of its length along the northern ridge of Double Oak Mountain. The White crosses Shackleford Point, which at 1,260 feet in altitude is the park's highest point. The White Trail traverses sandstone outcroppings and can be rocky in places, but it offers great views. At its southern end, the White Trail provides access to Peavine Falls and its parking lot. Nearer its northern end, the White passes through the popular forest crossroads known as Maggie's Glen.

BLUE TRAIL At 6.7 miles long, this trail steeply ascends Oak and Double Oak Mountains from the North Trailhead and quickly takes you to the more remote and scenic spots in the park, like the Eagle's Nest and King's Chair Overlooks. Once you top the mountain, the Blue Trail is relatively level as it travels parallel to the southern ridge of Double Oak Mountain, eventually reaching side trails to Peavine Gorge and Peavine Falls.

YELLOW TRAIL This trail doesn't climb to the park's highest points, but it's a workout nonetheless, as it continuously gains and loses elevation over the foothills between the North and South Trailheads. The Yellow Trail includes Maggie's Glen and a nice stretch along Lake Tranquility, also known as the Old Lake. The trail is 8 miles long from end to end.

GREEN TRAIL Starts from the South Trailhead and climbs steeply to Peavine Falls, about 2 miles. That's a lot of elevation gain in a short period. The best part of the Green Trail is the walk along the ridge after you cross the Red Trail; this segment offers nice views as well as connections to Peavine Falls.

TREETOP NATURE TRAIL This elevated boardwalk houses six cages with nonreleasable birds of prey. It starts across the street from the park headquarters on Double Oak Lake and connects to the Oak Mountain Interpretive Center.

ORANGE TRAIL For horses only. Throughout the park, everyone is supposed to yield to people on horseback.

Oak Mountain has a system of markers located every quarter-mile on its trails. The numbers on the markers don't repeat and offer a way for you to tell a park ranger where you are in case you get in trouble. They also allow you to compute mileage if you know the system: The Blue Trail starts at 1 and goes up to 26; the White starts at 27 in the south and goes to 51 in the north; the Green, 52 to 59; the Yellow, 60 to 86; and the Red, 100 to 160. Short connectors between the main trails allow for the creation of all sorts of route options.

More Information

DIRECTIONS: From Birmingham, take I-65 South to Exit 246. Turn right onto AL 119 at the end of the ramp, then take your first left onto Oak Mountain Park Road. Drive 2 miles to a four-way stop and take a left, following the signs into the park.

From US 280, take AL 119 South (toward Pelham) 6 miles and turn left onto Oak Mountain Park Road. Continue to the back entrance of the park, bearing left into the park.

ACCESS: Hours vary by season but are generally 7 a.m.–sunset; call for current hours. The front gate is open 24 hours for registered overnight guests. Day-use fees are $3 for adults, $1 for children ages 6–11 and adults age 62 and up. Yearly memberships are available.

MAPS: An excellent park map by Thigpen Designs is available on the website, at the entrances, at the park headquarters, and at the country store.

FACILITIES: Park headquarters is at 200 Terrace Dr. on Double Oak Lake. The Interpretive Center and Wildlife Rehabilitation Center are off Terrace Drive. Picnic areas can be found throughout the park. The Peavine Falls Parking Area and the North Trailhead have portable restrooms. Additional facilities are noted in the hikes that follow.

WHEELCHAIR ACCESS: The hikes in this chapter are not accessible, but the Treetop Nature Trail is.

COMMENTS: In warm weather, be cautious of snakes, ticks, poison ivy, and stinging insects. Overnight camping is permitted, though registration is required; no open campfires. Make sure that you have enough water for both you and your pets, if you bring them on the trails. Stay on trails. Be aware of the color-coded trail-marking system in case of emergency.

CONTACTS: 205-620-2520, **alapark.com/oakmountain.** For more information on the park's geology and biology, visit **trekbirmingham.com/places/oak-mountain-state-park.**

Oak Mountain State Park: King's Chair Loop

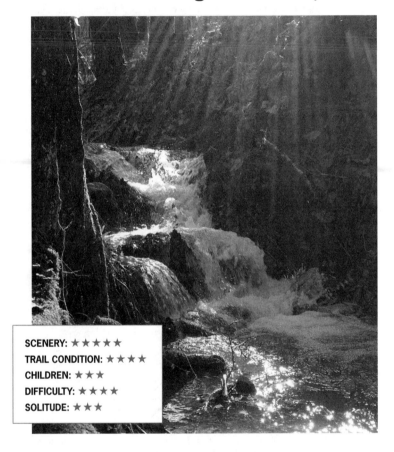

SCENERY: ★ ★ ★ ★ ★
TRAIL CONDITION: ★ ★ ★ ★
CHILDREN: ★ ★ ★
DIFFICULTY: ★ ★ ★ ★
SOLITUDE: ★ ★ ★

GPS TRAILHEAD COORDINATES: N33° 21.438' W86° 42.288'

DISTANCE & CONFIGURATION: 5-mile loop

HIKING TIME: 3 hours

HIGHLIGHTS: Challenging uphills, great mountaintop views from Eagle's Nest and King's Chair, wet-weather waterfalls

ELEVATION: 600' at trailhead, 1,200' at peak

ACCESS, MAPS, WHEELCHAIR ACCESS: See previous page.

FACILITIES: Restrooms and changing rooms at the trailhead

COMMENTS: Remember that the Red Trail is a shared hiking and mountain biking trail.

Overview

This route is intense because of its uphill climb and the scenic rewards it provides. It's a great hike for fall colors, providing sweeping scenic vistas. In wet weather, cascading streams tumble down the mountainside. In any season, it's a quick way to feel far from civilization.

From the North Trailhead, this hike follows the Blue Trail up Double Oak Mountain to two of the park's favorite overlooks. It continues southwest along the south rim of the mountain before taking the south Red–Blue Connector Trail to the Red Trail, which heads downhill back to the north trailhead.

Route Details

This hike doesn't mess around. It makes an immediate climb up Oak Mountain. Between the North Trailhead and the Eagle's Nest overlook there is a 500-foot elevation gain, and that's in the first mile and a half. But that early and intense exertion pays dividends. You get away from civilization quickly. Thanks to the size of the park and the way the trail twists up the ridges, you encounter views on this hike in which all you see is woods and mountains, quick access to the feeling that you've wandered off someplace remote.

We hiked parts of this route in the warm and dry early fall and enjoyed the way the breezes on the ridges cooled us after a tough climb. We returned in winter after a rain and were surprised to find that what had been dry drainages in the fall had become a series of gushing waterfalls. There was so much water that creek crossings on the Red Trail offered a challenge for anyone wanting to keep their feet dry.

The hike starts at the North Trailhead, across from the gravel parking lot on the north end of the park, near the lower lakes and the park entrance off AL 119.

While the White, Yellow, and Red Trails gain elevation gradually, the Blue Trail heads directly up the mountain. It is well marked, with plastic blue blazes nailed to trees. Distance markers are posted

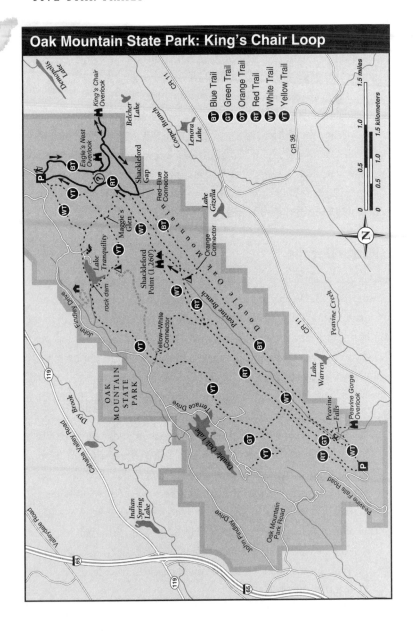

Oak Mountain State Park: King's Chair Loop

BT Blue Trail
GT Green Trail
OT Orange Trail
RT Red Trail
WT White Trail
YT Yellow Trail

every quarter-mile; on the Blue Trail, they start at zero and go up. So at Post 4, you've gone 1 mile.

The forests are a mix of pine and hardwood, with a nice sampling of longleaf pines on the ridges and white oaks in the draws; the latter provide a generous supply of fat acorns in the fall. When we went back in winter, the acorns were harder to find, likely gobbled up by the wintering wildlife. What was present in the winter that had not been there in the fall was water. And lots of it. A little less than a half-mile into the hike, you begin crossing a series of streams dropping down the mountainside, creating little waterfalls as they go. At the 1-mile mark, you pass the north Red–Blue Connector Trail, which serves as a shortcut back to the parking lot if you need it.

Shortly thereafter, the trail splits. Continuing straight, the original Blue Trail offers several unobstructed views of Shackleford Ridge, then descends gently to a saddle between ridges before resuming its upward climb. If you've had enough of steep hills by now, this is the way to go. Be forewarned, though, that heavy rains can turn the original Blue Trail into a swiftly flowing creek. Alternatively, if you turn left at the junction, a newer Blue Trail (with the same blue blazes) makes an exceedingly steep 0.2-mile climb to a rock outcropping at the Eagle's Nest overlook, then continues downhill not quite as precipitously to rejoin the original Blue Trail just before the final pitch up to the Double Oak Mountain ridgetop. From the top of the

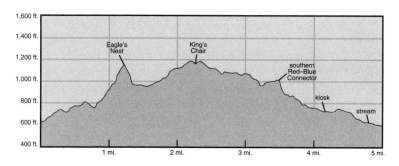

rock at Eagle's Nest, you can see yet another perspective of Shackleford Ridge and the park's highest point. From all points, your view is forest and twisting mountain ridges that hide any evidence of civilization.

At the 1.5-mile marker on the trail (you're about 2 miles into your hike if you went up to Eagle's Nest), you top the ridge and reach the junction with the spur trail to the King's Chair Overlook. Take the spur. At 0.3 mile, it's a little longer than the spur to Eagle's Nest, but it's much less arduous.

At the rocky outcropping of King's Chair, you get your first chance for wide-open views from the southeastern ridge of the mountain. In the far distance across the wide Coosa River Valley, the Talladega Mountain ridges are visible. In the middle distance, you'll see steam rising from the cooling towers at Alabama Power's Gaston electrical plant in south Shelby County, along the river.

Returning to the main trail, continue south along the ridge on the Blue Trail to the southern Red–Blue Connector. Take that connector, which cuts back to the north 0.75 mile to the Red Trail, which in turn takes you back to the North Trailhead. The return trip is especially nice if it has been raining. Those little mountain streams gather together with more volume, creating trailside waterfalls and challenging creek crossings. Along the way, you'll notice stonework in the drainage system along the road. In the 1930s, the Civilian Conservation Corps built the Red Road. Remember that you're sharing this trail with mountain bikers.

The trip back to the parking lot is well marked and easy.

Directions

From I-65, follow the directions on page 111. After entering the park, you'll drive almost its entire length to get to the North Trailhead.

From US 280, follow the directions on page 111. About a mile past the back entrance to the park, the North Trailhead parking lot will be on your right, along the main park road.

13

Oak Mountain State Park:
Lake Tranquility Loop

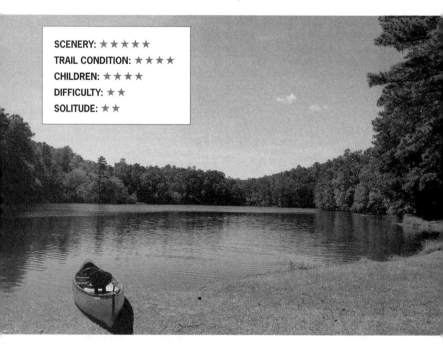

SCENERY: ★ ★ ★ ★ ★
TRAIL CONDITION: ★ ★ ★ ★
CHILDREN: ★ ★ ★ ★
DIFFICULTY: ★ ★
SOLITUDE: ★ ★

GPS TRAILHEAD COORDINATES: N33° 21.431' W86° 42.288'

DISTANCE & CONFIGURATION: 3.6-mile loop

HIKING TIME: 2.5 hours

HIGHLIGHTS: Abundant wildflowers and ferns, Maggie's Glen, Lake Tranquility

ELEVATION: Start at 600', climb to 800.5', descend to 554', and return to 600'.

ACCESS, MAPS, WHEELCHAIR ACCESS: See page 111.

FACILITIES: Restroom and changing room at the trailhead; table and benches at Maggie's Glen

COMMENTS: Lake Tranquility is partially ringed by rental cabins. Use of the lake is restricted to guests who've paid to rent those cabins. Respect their privacy.

Overview

This hike, which starts on the Yellow Trail and returns on the White, covers rolling, wooded terrain for the first mile and a half until it

Oak Mountain State Park: Lake Tranquility Loop

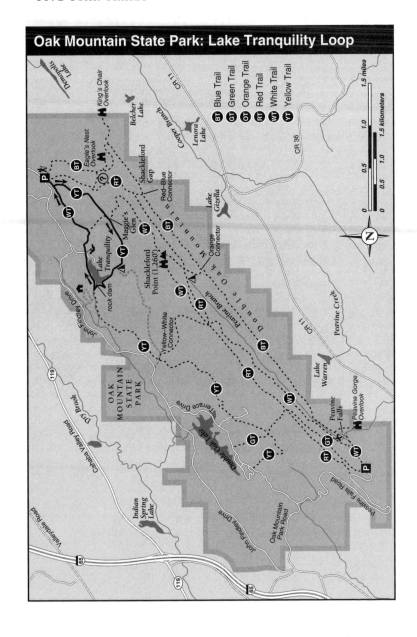

BT Blue Trail
GT Green Trail
OT Orange Trail
RT Red Trail
WT White Trail
YT Yellow Trail

1.5 miles
1.5 kilometers

reaches Maggie's Glen. A mile later, you reach the shores of Lake Tranquility. Circle it and make a connection across the rental-cabin access road to the White Trail, which returns to the North Trailhead.

Route Details

From the North Trailhead, walk down the Red Road about 50 yards and turn right at the sign that that reads MAGGIE'S GLEN 1.3 MILES. Not long thereafter, the White and Yellow Trails split—follow the Yellow Trail. For most of its course through the park, from the South Trailhead to the North, the Yellow Trail goes up and down. It never ascends the high ridges of Double Oak Mountain, but it does provide a vigorous walk in the foothills.

In this early stretch of trail, the forest is recovering from a pine beetle infestation. Thick patches of juvenile pine trees compete for sunlight; there are also a decent number of longleaf pines and saplings. In late September, the hike offered a wide variety of wildflowers. My daughter, Anna, worked the camera, and we took shots of everything we saw. I know a few flowers but not many. Though the colors were relatively consistent, in pinks, purples, yellows, and whites, the forms and combinations seemed unlimited.

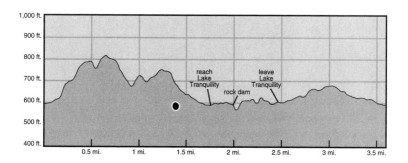

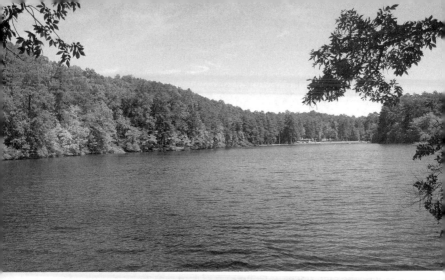

A VIEW FROM THE FAR END OF LAKE TRANQUILITY. GUESTS AT THE RENTAL CABINS CAN PADDLE AND FISH THIS LAKE TUCKED INTO THE MOUNTAINSIDE.

From the pine-topped hills, the trail drops steeply into Maggie's Glen, an open area by a creek where the White and Yellow Trails reconnect. It's a nice place for a picnic and a romp in the mossy green rocks.

The hike continues across the creek, heading up a little draw. The White Trail diverges to the left, uphill toward the heights of Double Oak Mountain. We stayed on the Yellow Trail, gaining elevation again and then dropping into a moist valley where another feeder creek drains toward Lake Tranquility. The park's No. 2–designated campsite is here. The trees here are well-watered and wide-trunked. Ferns, mosses, and mushrooms are abundant. Along this stretch and continuing once you get to the lake, you might notice some structures on the high ridges to your left (southwest). These were the original cabins built by the Civilian Conservation Corps during the Depression. The CCC also built the stone dam that you'll see a little farther on, the dam that makes Lake Tranquility, also known as Old Lake.

The rustic cabins had fallen into disrepair until local Boy Scout troops took an interest. A series of Eagle Scout projects has restored many of the cabins, which are once again used for Scout camping.

Before you actually emerge on the banks of the lake, you'll first see a swampy backwater formed by a beaver's dam. The 28-acre lake is cupped by the mountains and surrounded by dense forest. Turning left across a wooden bridge, the Yellow Trail travels along the lake's southwestern shore. The trailside is rich in wildflowers and ferns and offers several spots where you can look out over the expanse of lake and appreciate the timbered mountainsides or the fall colors, depending on the season. You may see people riding horses along this stretch.

As you make your way around the lake, you'll come upon the rock dam. Excess water spills over it and into a creek below. You'll see a dirt road on the opposite side of the dam—you want to get there. Follow the Yellow Trail as it crosses the dam and descends to the creek below. In drier times, it's easy to rock-hop across the creek and climb the opposite bank to the dirt road, but sometimes the water is high and there's really no good place to cross. In that case, follow the Yellow Trail another 0.1 mile and exit into the pavilion and picnic area. From there, turn right on the gravel road and continue past the BMX track to a small building with a soda machine. Walk downhill behind the building and you'll hook up with the dirt road.

Follow the dirt road along the creek and around the lake to the rental cabins. Go left on the paved road past a playground until you see a medium-sized rectangular building on the right. Turn right and pass the long side of the building to head into a grassy field. On the opposite side of the field, following white blazes, continue straight into the woods and intersect the main White Trail. Bear northeast for the final mile of the walk toward the trailhead and parking lot. This stretch of the White Trail follows a creek through a moist, low-lying valley. On our jaunt, we saw multiple varieties of colorful mushrooms. You'll reconnect to the Yellow Trail and retrace your path toward the parking lot.

Directions

From I-65, follow the directions on page 111. After entering the park, you'll drive almost its entire length to get to the North Trailhead.

From US 280, follow the directions on page 111. About a mile past the back entrance to the park, the North Trailhead parking lot will be on your right, along the main park road.

14

Oak Mountain State Park:
Peavine Falls

SCENERY: ★ ★ ★ ★ ★
TRAIL CONDITION: ★ ★ ★ ★
CHILDREN: ★ ★ ★ ★
DIFFICULTY: ★ ★
SOLITUDE: ★

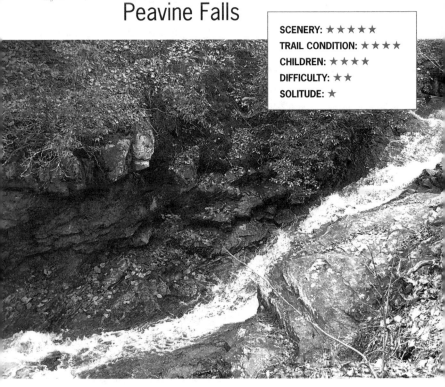

GPS TRAILHEAD COORDINATES: N33° 18.148' W86° 45.706'

DISTANCE & CONFIGURATION: 1 mile down and back (with suggested alternatives that can lengthen the hikes to 3 or 4 miles)

HIKING TIME: 1 hour (or you can easily make it a half-day outing)

HIGHLIGHTS: One large waterfall about 20 feet tall and several waterfalls and cascades below that; stands of longleaf pine

ELEVATION: 1,030' at start, 850' at the base of the falls

ACCESS, MAPS, WHEELCHAIR ACCESS: See page 111.

FACILITIES: Portable restrooms, a stone pavilion, and picnic tables at the Peavine Falls parking lot; information kiosk and benches along the route

COMMENTS: Though this hike is short, it's steep; some exertion is required. Watch your footing—rocks can be slippery. Keep an eye on kids around drops. The waterfall is somewhat rain-dependent. Don't expect much of a show in the heat of summer or during prolonged dry spells. The drive up to the Peavine Falls Parking Area is scenic, but the road is narrow and you should watch for bicyclists.

Overview

This is the classic family starter hike: a nice drive with spots along the way to stop and take in mountaintop views; a short, steep hike through longleaf pine down into a gorge rich with mountain laurel where you'll find the landmark waterfall. You'll see kids, couples, and retirees making this pilgrimage. With add-ons, you can crest Double Oak Mountain and explore a little history too.

Route Details

As I mentioned earlier, my first hike was to Peavine Falls. My parents took us. The part I remember most was the steep walk back to the parking lot. I was determined to make it without complaint, especially since my brother, three years younger than I, was complaining. In retrospect, he was 3 years old. I don't deserve the credit I was giving myself.

The direct venture to the falls is a round-trip of about a mile. But because you're losing about 200 feet in elevation and then gaining it back, it's a little more challenging than it sounds.

In a decently wet year and in the cooler months, you'll get a really pretty scene. Peavine Branch—so named because the mountain stream is as twisty as a pea vine—suddenly goes from a meandering creek down a drop of more than 20 feet. It then tumbles through cascades and chutes below that, losing a total of 65 feet of elevation. At the base of the first big falls are a pool and boulders to perch on as you ponder the rewards of getting away to this deep, sheltered canyon.

Don't expect to have it all to yourself; this is one secret place we all know about.

From the middle of the parking lot, a typical hiking trail descends to a bridge crossing Peavine Branch above the falls. A more mellow route to the same place is a gravel road to the right of the parking area that ultimately intersects the hiking trail 0.1 mile uphill of the bridge.

Oak Mountain State Park: Peavine Falls

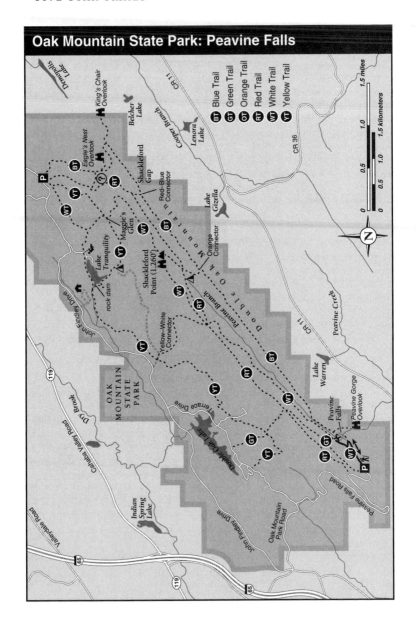

BT Blue Trail
GT Green Trail
OT Orange Trail
RT Red Trail
WT White Trail
YT Yellow Trail

All this is pretty straightforward, but as you approach the falls, your options multiply. There are official offshoot trails, unofficial off-shoots, and offshoots to offshoots, so it would be hard to provide clear instructions about how to get down to the base of the falls.

At the bridge that crosses Peavine Branch near the top of the falls, the White Trail heads upstream, away from the falls. But across that bridge are the Blue Trail and several options for descending to the bottom of the falls from the east side.

Whichever way you get there, enjoy yourself once you're down in the gorge. A short loop trail down either side of the creek is referred to as Falls Creek Loop, which offers more waterfalls and chutes. At the far end of the creek, you can cross and return via the opposite bank.

If you climb the eastern side of the gorge, once you reach the Blue Trail you can walk a little to the northeast (away from the parking lot) and find a spur trail to the Peavine Gorge Overlook. This trail heads south, staying up on the rim of Peavine Gorge, and offers pretty views, ending at the Rim Shelter overlook, 0.3 mile down the trail.

Returning to the bridge at the top of the falls, you have other options for adding some extra hiking to your visit. You can add a mile and a mountaintop moment by taking the White Trail upstream on the branch and then taking a left on the White–Green Connector. The first stretch along the creek is nice, with beech trees whose roots dip into the stream like overgrown drinking straws. The connector

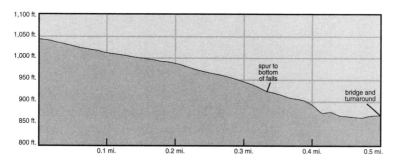

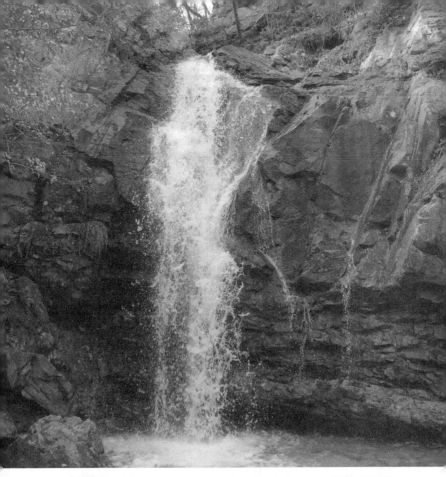

PEAVINE FALLS PUTS ON A SHOW IN THE RAINY SEASON. DOWNSTREAM FROM THE MAIN FALLS LIES A SERIES OF SMALLER FALLS AND CHUTES.

trail leaves the creek and climbs the ridge. When you intersect the Green Trail, take a left (heading southwest) and follow it up the ridge along sandstone outcroppings. The trail then loops back to the Peavine Falls parking lot. This climb adds about 75 extra feet of elevation gain and a feeling of accomplishment.

Another variation on the Peavine theme is to park at the Ada Overlook, on the pulloff before you get to the Peavine Falls Parking Area. This is the southern end of the Red Trail. There is an observation deck built there and parking. You're looking out over the Cahaba

Valley, which, despite all the development, is still wooded—except for the Galleria, of course. You have a nice view of it from up here.

To hike from here, you can take either the main Red Trail/Double Oak Trail or a parallel red trail called the CCC Fire Pits Trail. This weaves along the mountainside visiting a succession of stone fire pits built by those Depression-era crews that cut the first roads and built the first cabins in the park.

The Red Trail intersects the Green, which you take in the direction of the falls. Take the Green–White Connector to the White, then the White to the top of the falls. From there, get your Peavine fix, then either backtrack or take the White Trail to the Peavine parking lot, where you can access the Green Trail and shortly thereafter a Green–Red Connector that takes you back to the Ada Overlook. That's a loop of about 2.5 miles, excluding whatever exploring you do around Peavine Falls.

If you're making a simple out-and-back hike to the falls and you find yourself wanting a little more, you have several options. Before or after, stop at the **Oak Mountain Interpretive Center** for exhibits on the biology and geology of the park. Right next door to that is the **Alabama Wildlife Center,** where injured birds are rehabilitated. Along associated trails, you can see recovering wildlife in shelters. The Treetop Nature Trail, which begins near the South Trailhead and park headquarters and connects to the Wildlife and Interpretive Centers, offers some of these sights.

Directions

From I-65, follow the directions on page 111. To get to the Peavine Falls Parking Area, drive 2 miles past the park entrance and take a right onto Terrace Drive. Go past Double Oak Lake, the park headquarters, and the South Trailhead, continuing on Peavine Falls Road.

From US 280, follow the directions on page 111 to reach the back entrance of the park. Drive nearly the length of the park and take a left onto Terrace Drive. Continue on Terrace Drive, which becomes Peavine Falls Road.

Oak Mountain State Park:
Shackleford High Points Hike

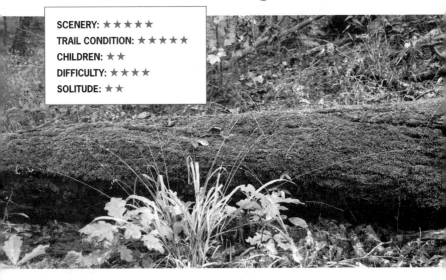

SCENERY: ★ ★ ★ ★ ★
TRAIL CONDITION: ★ ★ ★ ★ ★
CHILDREN: ★ ★
DIFFICULTY: ★ ★ ★ ★
SOLITUDE: ★ ★

GPS TRAILHEAD COORDINATES: N33° 21.431' W86° 42.288'

DISTANCE & CONFIGURATION: 7-mile loop

HIKING TIME: 5 hours

HIGHLIGHTS: Great climbs to rocky scenic overlooks from both sides of Double Oak Mountain; traverses the highest point in the park, Shackleford Point, and returns through Maggie's Glen

ELEVATION: 600' at North Trailhead, 1,260' at Shackleford Point

ACCESS, MAPS, WHEELCHAIR ACCESS: See page 111.

FACILITIES: Campsites and benches; restroom at trailhead

COMMENTS: If you plan to turn this into an overnight campout, pack in adequate water. The mountaintop streams are very rain-dependent.

Overview

This hike features segments of both the Blue and White Trails, traveling through the highest points in the park and offering great views along the way. It's a vigorous walk that can be done in one long day. There is also a primitive campsite along the way if you want to break it into two modest days.

Route Details

From the North Trailhead, start with the steep climb up the Blue Trail. For a detailed description of this portion of the hike, see Hike 12, King's Chair Loop (page 112). If you're trying to cover this loop in a single day, you might opt out of the side trips to Eagle's Nest and King's Chair, though they're worth the walk if you aren't carrying a pack.

Speaking of, coming up that Blue Trail with a loaded pack on your back is a challenge. My son James, 10 at the time, is a hearty and cheerful hiker, but by the time we reached the spur to King's Chair, a little over a mile in, he was worn out. With a little rest he was fine, especially since the rest of the trip is less challenge and more reward.

Once you've gained that initial 400 feet in elevation in the first mile, the remaining 100 feet of elevation gain is spread out and barely perceptible.

The segment of the Blue Trail beyond the King's Chair Overlook is one of my favorite stretches in the park, and probably the most remote and solitary. It's a pleasant forest walk under a mature tree canopy, with an understory of red maples. At the same time, you have numerous opportunities to walk out to the boulders that line the southern ridge of the mountain for sweeping views of the wooded expanses to the south.

From the King's Chair spur trail, you have about 2 miles to walk before you reach the Orange Connector, which you'll find 3.5 miles from the North Trailhead.

The Orange Connector takes you down a dip in the mountaintop and across to the White Trail and the north ridge of Double Oak Mountain, also known as Shackleford Ridge. Along this connector you'll find Oak Mountain's designated Primitive Campsite 3, complete with a fire ring. It's nice place to camp, but there is no water source nearby. Peavine Branch is marked on maps as originating there. We found the channel but found no water in it, despite some recent rains.

The Orange Connector crosses the Red Trail, which is a biking and hiking trail combined, so mind yourself.

Oak Mountain State Park: Shackleford High Points Hike

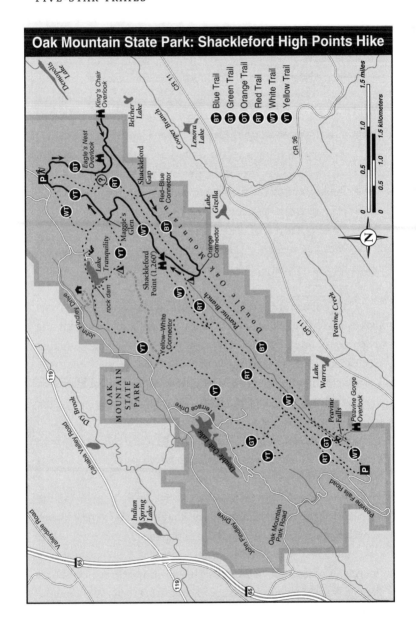

Blue Trail
Green Trail
Orange Trail
Red Trail
White Trail
Yellow Trail

You could turn north on the Red Trail here and head back to the parking lot, but you'd miss the hike to Shackleford Point, which, at 1,260 feet, is the highest point in the park. The White Trail along Shackleford Ridge offers great views to the north and west, including glimpses of the Riverchase Galleria shopping center. Much of the hike is along the sandstone outcropping of the ridge and is rocky, so a good pair of hiking boots comes in handy. That geology leads to smaller, stunted trees and open spaces. Along the trail are purple aster and goldenrod. When you round the ridge, you're looking across Shackleford Gap at the trail you mounted earlier in the day, the overlook near Eagle's Nest.

The White Trail then descends, switching back and forth down the mountainside. At the intersection with the Yellow Trail, take a right (northwest) toward Maggie's Glen, which you reach in a short while. Leaving Maggie's Glen, take the Yellow Trail toward the parking lot.

Directions

From I-65, follow the directions on page 111. After entering the park, you'll drive almost its entire length to get to the North Trailhead.

From US 280, follow the directions on page 111. About a mile past the back entrance to the park, the North Trailhead parking lot will be on your right, along the main park road.

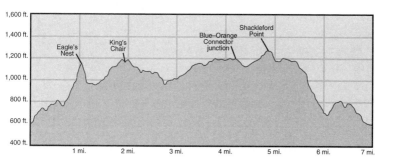

Red Mountain Park (Hikes 16–18)

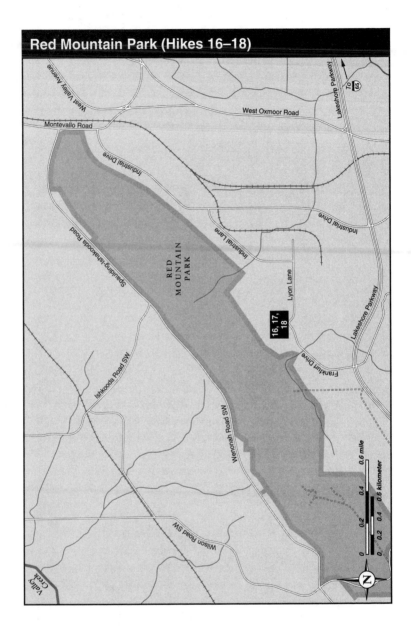

Red Mountain Park

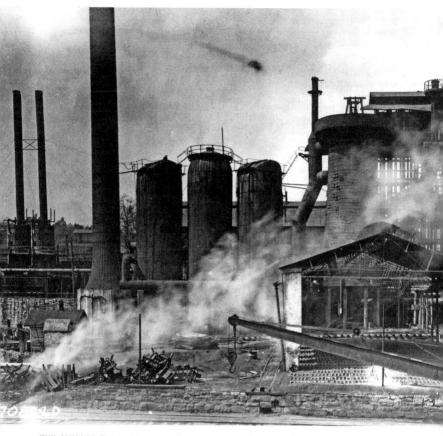

THE OXMOOR FURNACE, ON SHADES CREEK, WAS FED BY IRON ORE MINED FROM WHAT IS NOW RED MOUNTAIN PARK.
Photo: Birmingham, Ala., Public Library Archives

Red Mountain Park Overview

THE YOUNGEST, BIGGEST, AND MOST DYNAMIC hiking destination in Birmingham also happens to be where the city, or at least its original essential industry, began. The first commercial ore mine in the Birmingham District was dug in what is now Red Mountain Park to supply the Civil War–era Oxmoor Furnace.

The park opened to the public in 2012 after the community gathered $7 million through a mix of charitable contributions and public money to purchase the 4-mile-long strip of Red Mountain from U.S. Steel at a discount.

Thickets of privet and kudzu have been hacked away so visitors can walk again on what was the initial segment of the Birmingham Mineral Railroad, a network of tracks begun in the 1880s that would become the industrial bloodstream of the iron-and-steel industry.

It's hard to imagine that at the beginning of the 20th century, Red Mountain was shorn of timber, punctuated by numerous ore mines, and crisscrossed with rail lines. As the 21st century gathers steam, that same mountainside supports a reborn forest where the trees have been hung with zip lines and the hillsides laced with hiking and biking trails. Where tipples once loaded ore trains, tree houses now stand on the ridges overlooking the valley.

Red Mountain Park comprises 1,500 acres west of I-65 and the Wildwood development off Lakeshore Parkway. As of December 2014, the park will have nearly 15 miles of trails open to hikers, runners, and bikers. Further connections are under construction, including a trail along a railroad high line that runs above the street grid from the edge of the park toward Midfield and Fairfield. In 2014, the park also added the 6-acre Remy's Dog Park and the 80-foot Kaul Adventure Tower, a climbing and rappelling tower that is also the base for a 1,600-foot zip line, a new companion to the existing Red Ore Zip Tour.

The park is supported through donations and through revenue generated by the zip-line courses and the Hugh Kaul Beanstalk Forest, an obstacle challenge in the trees.

I have a particular affection for Red Mountain Park because I started exploring it when the park was just being proposed. We went out to visit Ervin Batain, an enterprising and eccentric resident of a neighborhood that had once been the Ishkooda mining camp. Batain had set up a makeshift mining museum, The 3D/No. 11 Mining Camp & Nature Trail, in back of his house.

He blazed a trail that led up Red Mountain to the ruins of U.S. Steel's iron ore mine and up to the ridge road, where it intersected what today is the park's Redding–Ishkooda Trail. It's a spot where you're atop the ridge and sheltered by pine trees, where there always seems to be a breeze. When I reached that peaceful place the first time, I remember hoping that others could share that experience. Every time I walk through that corridor again, I feel a little thrill as I fast-forward through what's happened since.

The park is owned by the state and managed by an appointed commission. Its operations receive no regular stream of taxpayer dollars. It's been built through grants, donations, volunteerism, and entrepreneurship.

Red Mountain offers a variety of trails. Wide paths follow old rail beds, and singletrack trails slither through the draws on the mountain flanks. The trails are dotted with industrial archaeological sites: old mine entrances, stone supports for ore-loading structures, and the remains of buildings. In some places the forest feels primeval, as if you're seeing the original landscape. In other spots you realize that the mountain has been radically reshaped and altered, and that invasive kudzu and privet block out the native flora.

Wherever you turn and whenever you visit, there is something new to discover, whether something natural brought on by the change in the seasons or something man-made, recently uncovered, or newly built as the park grows and evolves.

Trailhead

Red Mountain Park's central trailhead is located at 2011 Frankfurt Drive, off Lakeshore Parkway (see Directions, page 137). A neighborhood trailhead is under development on the north side of the mountain off Venice Road.

Trails

From the parking lot, cross Lyon Lane and follow the signs to the trails. You'll first walk up a gravel entrance road for about 0.2 mile before reaching an information kiosk, where park maps are available. A small donation is requested in exchange for a map (keep in mind that the park receives no taxpayer support for operations). Facing the kiosk, the **Birmingham Mineral Railroad (BMRR) South Trail** (1.7 miles) heads off to your left (southwest). The flat and wide trail follows the path of what was a rail line serving mines on the south (Shades Valley) side of the mountain. At its western end is the most intact structure on the property: the hoist house that served the mine at Redding, a long-vanished community located around that mine near present-day Venice Road. On the north (Jones Valley) side of the mountain runs the **BMRR North Trail** (0.6 mile), which is similar in character and which served the mines on the Birmingham side of the mountain, connecting them to the mills and furnaces in the valley.

The **Redding–Ishkooda Trail** (3.1 miles) climbs from the Redding Shaft Mine at the western end of the developed park site to the top of the Red Mountain ridge, following the ridge all the way out to the northeastern end of the park to the city overlook at Grace's Gap. The terrain and character of this trail vary: Some of the trail follows a rail bed; other sections are singletrack. Along the way are stops at overlooks and three tree houses.

The **TCI Connector Trail** (0.63 mile), a wide gravel road, runs from the BMRR South to the BMRR North. While it does go up and over the ridge, it's at a gentle grade, passing the zip-line course along the way.

The steep, singletrack **Smythe Trail** (0.53 mile) also connects the BMRR South with the BMRR North by hiking straight up Red Mountain. Reaching the ridge, it briefly runs east in conjunction with the Redding–Ishkooda Trail before dropping off the ridge and connecting on the Jones Valley side of the mountain with the BMRR North

Trail. The Smythe serves as a shortcut to the ridge for a visit to the SkyHy Treehouse (2.4 miles out-and-back) or the Ishkooda Overlook (a little more than 2 miles out-and-back).

The **Songo Trail** (9.42 miles) is a singletrack shortcut through the woods up the ridge from the Redding Shaft Mine to the Redding–Ishkooda Trail at the SkyHy Treehouse.

The **Ike Maston Trail** (2.5 miles) is a singletrack trail running northeast–southwest, connecting the three mine portals on the Shades Valley side of the mountain, starting with Ishkooda No. 14, then Ishkooda No. 13, and all the way out to the Redding Mine. It's named for the late Ike Maston, a retired ore miner who helped create a picture of life in the park through the Red Mountain Park Oral History Project. Along the way, the Maston Trail winds in and out of the draws on the mountainside, gaining and losing elevation. End-to-end, it's a tough walk, but it's a less-traveled path with some very pretty sections of woods.

The singletrack **Eureka Mines Trail** (0.55 mile) leaves from the main kiosk and heads into the woods, tracing the edge of a stone quarry. That trail skirts the adventure course area on the way to the No. 13 Mine, where it intersects the Ike Maston Trail. Branching off is a spur to the No. 14 Mine.

More Information

DIRECTIONS: From I-65, take Exit 255 onto Lakeshore Parkway and head west for 3 miles; turn right onto Frankfurt Drive. As you approach the cul-de-sac that is the end of Frankfurt Drive, veer sharply right onto Lyon Lane and follow the signs into the gravel parking lot. Coming from Bessemer, Frankfurt Drive is 6 miles east of Lakeshore Parkway's intersection with AL 150.

ACCESS: March–October, 7 a.m.–7 p.m.; November–February, 7 a.m.–7 p.m. Admission is free, but consider donating and/or joining the volunteer and support organization **The Friends of Red Mountain Park (friendsofredmountainpark.org)**.

MAPS: An excellent park map is available at **redmountainpark.org;** mouse over "Park Overview" and choose "The Trails of Red Mountain Park" from the pop-up menu.

FACILITIES: There are portable toilets in the area of the main kiosk, at the Redding Hoist House, and at the adventure area. Picnic tables and benches are deployed in various spots. There are also pet-waste stations in strategic locations—please pick up after your pooch. A ranger is always on duty to help guests.

WHEELCHAIR ACCESS: Both BMRR trails are accessible for wheelchairs fitted with off-road tires.

COMMENTS: Red Mountain was extensively mined and quarried. Stay on the trails. Watch out for cliffs, dropoffs, and areas of subsidence. Known mine entrances on the mountain are sealed, but if you discover one that isn't, stay out.

CONTACTS: 205-202-6043, **contact@redmountainpark.org**. Visit **redmountainpark.org** for more information or to book a zip-line tour or Beanstalk Forest adventure. Park ranger: 205-266-6000. Adventure area: 205-913-7899. For more information on the geology, ecology, and history of the mountain, visit **trekbirmingham.com/places/red-mountain-park.**

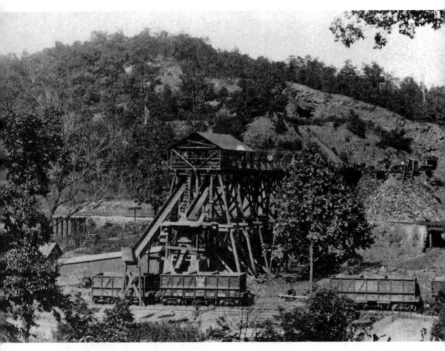

THE SPAULDING MINE (PICTURED CIRCA 1900) WAS LOCATED ACROSS GRACE'S GAP FROM WHAT IS NOW RED MOUNTAIN PARK.
Photo: Birmingham, Ala., Public Library Archives

16

Red Mountain Park:
Birmingham Mineral
Railroad Loop

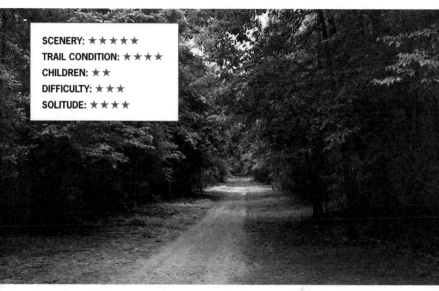

SCENERY: ★ ★ ★ ★ ★
TRAIL CONDITION: ★ ★ ★ ★
CHILDREN: ★ ★
DIFFICULTY: ★ ★ ★
SOLITUDE: ★ ★ ★ ★

GPS TRAILHEAD COORDINATES: N33° 26.882' W86° 51.765'

DISTANCE & CONFIGURATION: 4.5-mile loop

HIKING TIME: 3 hours

HIGHLIGHTS: Walk the historic path of the Birmingham Mineral Railroad (BMRR), once the bloodstream of Birmingham's iron-and-steel industry. Glimpse the remnants of mining structures along the way, including the oddly elegant Redding Hoist House. Gradually climb the mountain for views from the ridgetop and forest solitude, then descend to the northern flank of the mountain for more mining ruins, red rocks, and oakleaf hydrangeas.

ELEVATION: 700' at the start, 930' at the peak

ACCESS, MAPS, FACILITIES, WHEELCHAIR ACCESS: See pages 137–138.

COMMENTS: If you want a less taxing hike, you can travel out the BMRR South Trail to the Redding Shaft Mine, see the hoist house, and turn around. That would be a 2.5-mile out-and-back walk.

Overview

This is an ambitious hike when it comes to length, but it shows off many of the highlights of the park. It's a great route for runners, as

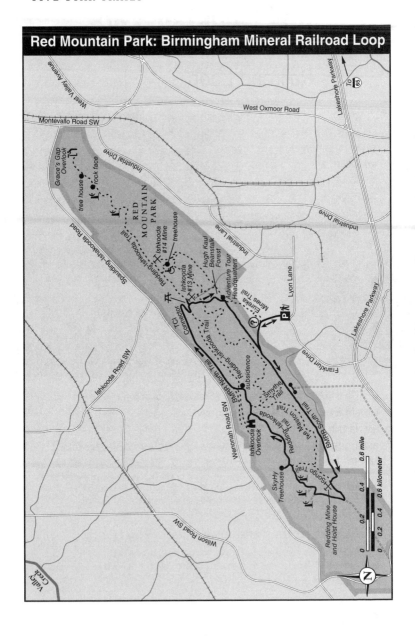

Red Mountain Park: Birmingham Mineral Railroad Loop

it follows the BMRR on the south and north sides of the mountain, on wide old rail beds that are straight and mostly flat. These railroad stretches are connected by the mildly challenging uphill of the Redding–Ishkooda Trail, which takes you up and over Red Mountain. After linking with the BMRR on the north flank of the mountain, the TCI Connector Trail leads you back over the ridge and down to the kiosk again. This is also a good workout on a mountain bike, with some physical demands on the uphills but not a lot in the way of daunting technical challenge.

Route Details

After you park and walk into the woods along a short gravel entrance road, you come to the main kiosk. Here you'll find maps and other information about the park.

Stand facing that kiosk and look to your right or left. The wide, straight gravel path, which runs from northeast to southwest at the base of this southern slope of Red Mountain, was the original Birmingham Mineral Railroad. This segment was part of the first 4 miles of track opened in 1884, connecting the Red Mountain mines to the main L&N line at Grace's Gap, near the northeast boundary of the park.

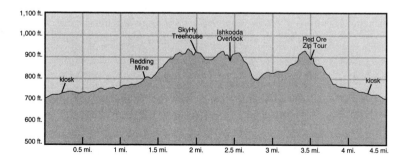

The BMRR would go on to loop the mountain and extend its tentacles to mines all over the district. There are stretches of the railroad at Ruffner Mountain Nature Preserve. It's been paved at the foot of Vulcan to form the Vulcan Trail. When it operated at its greatest extent, the BMRR was a network of 156 miles connecting industrial operations to the veins of red ore in and below Red Mountain.

Head west along the BMRR South Trail. As you proceed, keep in mind that this was once a busy rail corridor. You'll also be walking through areas that were once the mining communities of Smythe and Redding, villages where miners lived but which have long since vanished. Forests have grown in their place.

As you look into the woods, you'll also notice the invasive evergreen shrub privet on either side of the path, skulking at the edge of the woods. When this land was acquired from U.S. Steel, this corridor, particularly the portion after the pipeline crossing, had grown so thick with the Asian shrub that it was impassable.

Starting in the late 1800s, privet spread around the South as a popular landscaping hedge. Then it went wild. Privet produces berries. Birds eat the berries and then deposit the seeds elsewhere. Privet finds its way to pretty much any open space where the land has been disturbed. Once it takes root, it's hard to kill. Privet loved the rail corridors on Red Mountain. Feel free to take a sample.

As you proceed even farther west, you'll start noticing kudzu, another imported species. Back in the 1930s, kudzu was thought to be a great solution to stop erosion. It was apparently planted at mine sites up and down Red Mountain. Between the privet and the kudzu, whole worlds here on the mountain were consumed and lost to memory but are slowly being rediscovered. At least being lost helped protect what remained.

One such rediscovered jewel is the hoist house at the Redding Mine. At the yellow chain that marks the current end of the BMRR South Trail, take a right toward Red Mountain and follow the path, past the wetlands into an open area. Here you'll find a concrete pad and foundations and, above and beyond those, a large Spanish

Mission–style building: the hoist house, perched on a little rise. Near that building is an information display that will help you reconstruct how this operation worked. I'll try the basics: Beneath that concrete pad is a vertical mine shaft that drops deep below the surface to the iron seam that extends out under Shades Valley. A huge winch lodged in the hoist house pulled skips loaded with iron ore up from the bowels of the earth. These skips were dumped into a crusher, and then the ore was loaded on train cars to be hauled away.

After being acquired from Tutwiler Coal, Coke & Iron Company, this site was developed by Woodward Iron Company. Rick Woodward, the chairman of the company, was also the owner of the Birmingham (Coal) Barons baseball team and the builder of Rickwood Field, now known as America's oldest ballpark. His magnificent villa atop Red Mountain serves as the president's mansion for the University of Alabama at Birmingham. If you head back here, you'll have taken a 2.5-mile out-and-back walk.

To continue, you can take a shortcut through the woods up the Songo Trail. It connects to the Redding–Ishkooda Trail up on the ridge at the SkyHy Treehouse. For a longer hike, try the Redding–Ishkooda, which heads west from the hoist house. Shortly thereafter, it connects with a jeep road, then cuts back to the right (northeast) and climbs the hill. This ascent offers nice views of Shades Valley.

The stretch along the ridgetop is one of my favorites. The SkyHy Treehouse is fun: a swinging bridge out to a platform high above the valley with good views in the winter. But beyond that are some nice wooded spots where you're enfolded in the mountain. A breeze always seems to be blowing through the pines, and the only noise you tend to hear from civilization is the faraway train whistle.

As the trail continues, you again cross that open area, which is a pipeline corridor, only this time you're at the top of the ridge. Make sure to take a side trip to the Ishkooda Overlook on the Jones Valley (Birmingham) side of the mountain. It's by no means a pristine view: You're right above a gasoline-tank farm. Still, it's pretty. If you look carefully, you can see the old smokestacks of the Ensley Works steel plant, and on a clear day you can see the steam rising from the cooling towers at Alabama Power's Miller electrical plant.

A little farther down the ridge, you take a left as the trail leads downhill. On the right of that trail you'll see a little fenced-off area around some rocks. Look over the fence and you'll see a hole in the ground. On a hot day, if you hold your hand over the hole, you'll feel cool air coming out of the earth. This is a subsidence connected with one of the underground mines. It's neat, but it's also a good place for a reminder: Stay on the trails. These openings can form anywhere on the mountain, and you could fall into one by accident. And you don't want to end up in the mountain's maze of mines.

You'll have the option of taking a right and continuing to follow the Redding–Ishkooda Trail. Take that stretch one day. It's twisty and woodsy, with interesting rock formations. Redbuds bloom in the spring along here. However, if I'm ambling or jogging, I like to continue on to the BMRR North Trail, which is just downhill. When you reach it, turn right (northeast).

This is the mineral railroad on the north slope, and it's a little easier to imagine how the trains running along here were loaded. Mine skips were pulled up from underground, brought to the top of the mountain, and emptied into structures that allowed the ore to then be loaded onto the passing trains.

Ruins of those old loading structures dot this mountain slope. What's also found here, though, is a profusion of ferns and oakleaf hydrangeas, the state wildflower. It's a real credit to the resilience of these lovely plants that they recolonized this difficult terrain. Unfortunately, they face competition from privet and another Asian shrub that's taking over the woods, thorny elaeagnus.

The trail begins climbing the mountain, and you leave the BMRR North Trail to join the TCI Connector Trail, which takes you back over the mountain to the BMRR South Trail. As you walk, you'll notice outcroppings of the reddish, iron-tinged rock that gives the mountain its name. When you come to a large open area with picnic tables, you can again get your bearings from the informational displays provided. The

Redding–Ishkooda Trail reconnects here. And if you take a detour to the east on that trail, you can see the cut in the mountain where loads of ore were pulled up from the No. 13 Mine and the base of the mountain, up and over to be loaded on the railroad.

Continuing down the TCI Connector Trail, you'll be able to see the Red Ore Zip Tour on your left. There the trail splits about halfway down the mountain. Either choice is fine. You'll find your way back. But if you continue on the TCI Connector, remember this: When you reconnect to the BMRR South Trail, turn back left (northeast) to get back to the main kiosk. It always goes against my sense of direction.

Directions

See page 137.

17

Red Mountain Park:
Grace's Gap

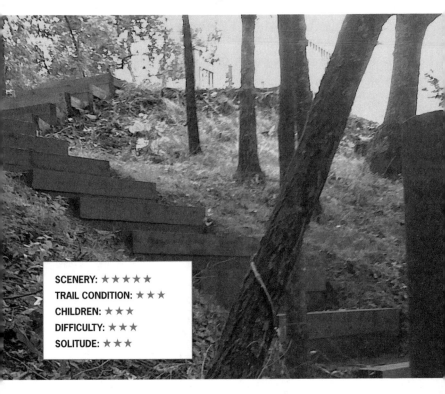

SCENERY: ★ ★ ★ ★ ★
TRAIL CONDITION: ★ ★ ★
CHILDREN: ★ ★ ★
DIFFICULTY: ★ ★ ★
SOLITUDE: ★ ★ ★

GPS TRAILHEAD COORDINATES: N33° 26.882' W86° 51.765'

DISTANCE & CONFIGURATION: 4.4-mile out-and-back

HIKING TIME: 2.5 hours

HIGHLIGHTS: Woods walk along the edge of a sandstone quarry, with views of the Red Ore Zip Tour and the Hugh Kaul Beanstalk Forest; gentle climb up Red Mountain. Along the ridge you'll find rock formations, ferns, and hydrangeas, plus two tree houses, one wheelchair-accessible, the other with an extended swinging bridge. At the far end, you reach the city overlook and observation deck at Grace's Gap.

ELEVATION: 700' at the start, 956' at the peak

ACCESS, MAPS: See page 137.

FACILITIES: Picnic tables at the quarry, upon reaching the ridge, and out at Grace's Gap

WHEELCHAIR ACCESS: An off-road wheelchair should be able to handle the trail as far as the Riley's Roost Treehouse. Beyond that, some trail sections become steep and rugged.

Overview

Your ultimate destination is the overlook at Grace's Gap, the far eastern end of Red Mountain Park. From here, you can see the mountain gap where the first commercial ore mining took place and look out to the city in Jones Valley that sprang up as a result of that mining and metal making. You make a gentle climb up Red Mountain and then take a level walk out on the ridge, past remnant red rocks and the ruins of mountaintop mining operations. Along the way are views of forested draws on the south side of the mountain.

Route Details

From the main kiosk, this hike follows the Eureka Mines Trail to the headquarters for the adventure course, then takes the TCI Connector up the ridge to the Redding–Ishkooda Trail. It then follows the Redding–Ishkooda northeast to Grace's Gap. This is a long hike, but the elevation gain is gradual. Once you reach the ridgetop, the trail is relatively level.

Because the first segment, along the Eureka Mines Trail, overlaps with ground covered by the Mine History Hike, I'll refer you there (see page 151) for a more complete description of the history of the area. Just enjoy the walk through the woods to the headquarters of the adventure course.

Once there, watch for adults and children frolicking up in the trees, and listen for the whiz of the zip lines. Consider a return visit for an afternoon on either the Zip Tour or the Beanstalk Forest. The Zip Tour is more of a guided thrill ride, a Peter Pan flight through the canopy. The Beanstalk Forest is self-guided and offers both mental and physical challenges as you balance, climb, and swing yourself from platform to platform. These attractions do cost money, but consider it an investment in fun and in the park: Though owned by the public, Red Mountain Park doesn't receive a regular stream of taxpayer support.

From the adventure area, the TCI Connector Trail climbs the mountain at a relatively gentle grade, switching back along the way.

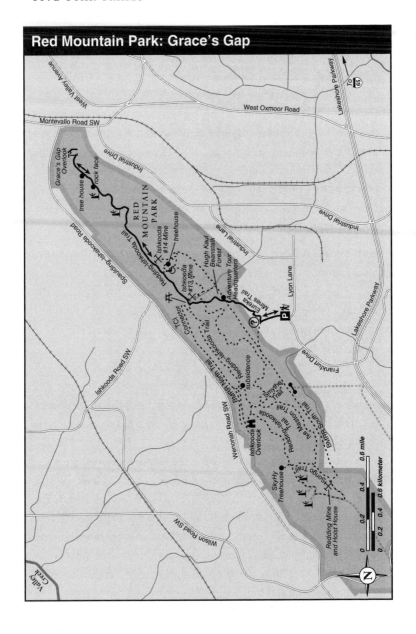

Red Mountain Park: Grace's Gap

If you haven't noticed already, you'll definitely notice the red in Red Mountain on this stretch. The tinge of iron can be seen in the rocks and the earth itself.

Near the mountaintop, you come to an open area and a junction of trails. You can stop here and look at the large map and historical photos posted there. On the southeast side of the trail are the foundations of what was a large machine shop. Heading northeast on the Redding–Ishkooda Trail, you cross a steep channel running up and down the mountain. Down this cut, at the base of the mountain on the Shades Valley side, was U.S. Steel's Ishkooda No. 13 Mine.

Skips loaded with ore were pulled out from underground up and over the mountain here. On the other side, the ore was loaded onto trains on the Birmingham Mineral Railroad for the journey to U.S. Steel's plants in Fairfield and Ensley.

As you proceed out the ridge, you'll see other building foundations, bolts bored into rocks, square-cut rock forms, and other evidence of how extensively the land has been reshaped and sculpted here.

This ridgetop route has been reopened only in the past couple of years. Along much of the route, privet, an invasive Asian shrub, had grown impenetrably thick. The war to push it back has continued along the ridge, with each advance against the privet revealing some new ruin previously hidden and preserved by the jungle.

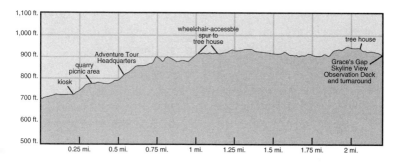

About 1 mile from the main kiosk, you'll find a detour to the right (the Shades Valley side). This large foundation is what is left of a bathhouse where miners could clean up after work before returning to their homes on the north side of the mountain. On the far side of the bathhouse foundations, the park has built a wheelchair-accessible tree house, Riley's Roost, that allows you to roll off level ground and out to a tree growing up from the ridge below. If you can see through the leaves to the valley below, you should be able to spot the remains of the Ishkooda No. 14 Mine, also on the Shades Valley side.

Continuing out the ridge, you'll proceed straight across a gravel access road that leads up to some transmission towers. The trail narrows and becomes slightly more irregular, with steps to climb and roots to avoid tripping on. There are also nice rock formations, ferns, and hydrangeas along this stretch. At about 2 miles from the main kiosk, you come to the second tree house, Rushing Rendezvous. This one is on the Jones Valley side of the mountain. Enjoy the long traverse of the swinging bridge out to this platform mounted high in an oak tree. In the late spring and summer, you can just glimpse civilization in the valley below.

Continuing on the trail to its end, you get a wide-open view of the city at the final observation deck at Grace's Gap. Red Mountain falls away at this point before rising again to the northeast.

The gap was named for Bayliss Earle Grace, who owned the land and farmed there until it was purchased in 1862 for the first commercial mining and metal-making enterprise in Birmingham (see the next hike for more details). It was through Grace's Gap that the L&N passed to reach what would become Birmingham.

After you've taken in the view and are ready to head back, you can explore a secondary trail that moves along the Jones Valley side of the ridge. After a short distance, it reconnects to the main trail.

Retrace your path to the parking lot. If you have weary and complaining troops, remind them that it's downhill going back.

Directions

See page 137.

18

Red Mountain Park:
Mine History Hike

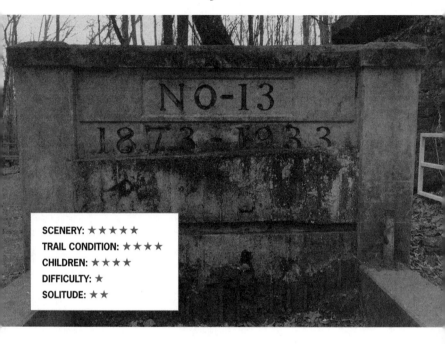

SCENERY: ★ ★ ★ ★ ★
TRAIL CONDITION: ★ ★ ★ ★
CHILDREN: ★ ★ ★ ★
DIFFICULTY: ★
SOLITUDE: ★ ★

GPS TRAILHEAD COORDINATES: N33° 26.882' W86° 51.765'

DISTANCE & CONFIGURATION: 1.5-mile out-and-back (option for a 2.5-mile loop)

HIKING TIME: 2 hours

HIGHLIGHTS: A woodland walk along the path of an early tramway to some of the oldest mines on Red Mountain. Glimpse the park's adventure area along the way.

ELEVATION: 700' to begin, 890' at the high point

ACCESS, MAPS, FACILITIES, WHEELCHAIR ACCESS: See page 137–138.

Overview

This hike follows the Eureka Mines Trail from the main kiosk to the sealed mouth (or portal) of the Ishkooda No. 13 Mine. Standing at the filled-in mine entrance, you can start to imagine what mining on the mountain looked like and appreciate the monumental nature of these enterprises. From here, you either return the way you came in

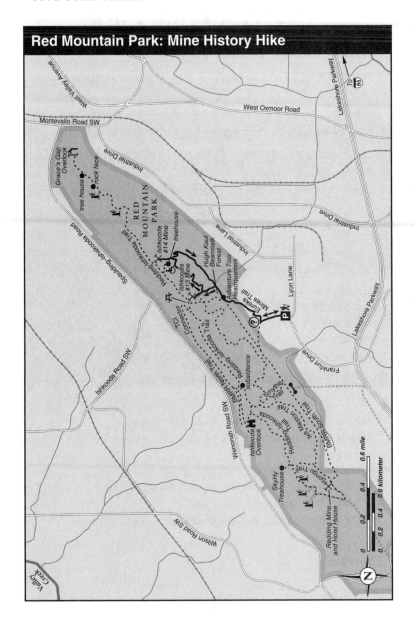

Red Mountain Park: Mine History Hike

or, for a longer hike, continue northeast on the Ike Maston Trail to the Ishkooda No. 14 Mine. From there, you can return via the No. 14 Mine Spur and the BMRR South Trail.

Route Details

Beginning in 1863, when the first commercial mine opened on Red Mountain, and continuing into the 1960s, miners removed more than 300 million tons of iron ore from mines that tunneled hundreds of feet into the mountain. Eventually an interconnected maze of mines spread out like a spiderweb beneath Shades Valley, with tunnels that reached all the way to the foot of Shades Mountain. Over the course of a century, mines on Red Mountain supplied on average 10% of the nation's iron ore.

This hike heads into the area of that first mining operation. In 1862, John T. Milner and Frank Gilmer used cash on loan from the Confederacy to launch the Red Mountain Iron and Coal Company. They bought 7,340 acres, including the area known as Grace's Gap, named for Bayliss Earle Grace, who had a farm there.

Ore dug from that early mining operation, which came to be known as Eureka No. 1, was hauled by wagon to the Oxmoor Furnace, which the company built on the banks of nearby Shades Creek. The Oxmoor Furnace, 31 feet tall and made of sandstone, went into

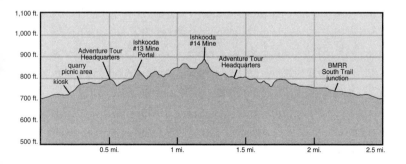

blast in 1863. According to *The Birmingham District: An Industrial History and Guide,* 60 men worked the furnace while an additional 200–300 slaves dug ore and cut and hauled wood to keep the furnace in blast. The furnace produced about 5–6 tons of iron a day. This iron, plus iron produced upstream on Shades Creek at the Irondale Furnace (see Hike 6), was hauled by wagon down Montevallo Road. Once it reached Montevallo, it was loaded onto a train that carried it to the Confederate arsenal at Selma.

That all came to an end on March 30, 1865, when Union troops swept through Shades Valley and destroyed the Oxmoor and Irondale Furnaces.

The furnace and mining operations were reopened in the 1870s by Daniel Pratt and Henry DeBardeleben. The revived enterprise connected Eureka No. 1 and a new mine, Eureka No. 2, with a tramway that also ran to the rebuilt furnace.

As you leave the main kiosk, follow the Eureka Mines Trail into the woods. This is the same route you take if you're heading toward the adventure course and zip line. After entering the woods, the trail climbs a rise and then proceeds along a little ridge. Portions of this trail follow that 1870s tramway. Right up that rise, a spur trail leads to a picnic area.

This picnic area, built by Boy Scouts, sits in what was a sandstone quarry. As you proceed along the Eureka Mines Trail, the quarry is in the woods to the right of the trail. The rock dug here was used to build the foundations of mining structures. Had I not been told, however, I never would have known what I was looking at—now all you see is forest covering some mildly unusual topography.

After a short hike, you come to the headquarters of the Hugh Kaul Beanstalk Forest and the Red Ore Zip Tour. If you're interested in riding or climbing in the tree canopy, make a reservation at the Red Mountain Park website. Or if you have a sudden urge to zip or climb, you can ask. Sometimes they can fit in a walk-up or two.

Continue on the Eureka Mines Trail south of the Beanstalk Forest. Follow signs to the No. 13 Mine. The trail will take you up a draw along a drainage on the eastern edge of the adventure course.

As you make your way toward the mine portal, you'll likely see some privet on the trailside. When the park was first acquired, this draw was a dense jungle of privet. I was part of a party of volunteers who cleared the initial path to this portal, which at the time was completely hidden.

It took me several visits and more clearing of the area to understand what I was looking at. This is the entrance to what was originally a Eureka mine. Later, under the ownership of U.S. Steel, it was renamed Ishkooda No. 13. Mines were numbered, rising numerically from west to east.

Ishkooda was a district on the mountain that ran from Grace's Gap to near present-day Venice Road, where another district, Wenonah, began. The Ishkooda mining camp, on the north side of the mountain, was built by the Tennessee Coal, Iron and Railroad Company, the mining and iron giant that was eventually purchased in 1907 by U.S. Steel. Ishkooda, situated along present-day Spaulding–Ishkooda Road, included housing built for miners, a company commissary, a church, a medical clinic, a community center, and a school.

If you're facing the portal, imagine following the slant of the hillside behind you through the portal and underground. Imagine tracks running down and carts loaded with ore being pulled up that incline from deep beneath the earth.

As it functioned in later years, once those carts were at the surface they would continue to be pulled up the mountain and over to be loaded onto the Birmingham Mineral Railroad (BMRR) running on the north side of the mountain. Earlier mining operations would have hauled the iron out to the south. A last word about a key piece of history tied to this site: Birmingham was founded in 1871, on the prospect of building a great industrial city on the basis of its natural resources. But in 1873, a financial panic and a cholera epidemic nearly ended the city before it began.

Thus, the 1873 date that's etched into the No. 13 mine portal is important. The mines here and the rebuilt furnaces at Oxmoor were the first major industrial venture in the district. In 1876, the Oxmoor Furnace conducted the first successful experimental run of iron using locally produced coke (coal from which the impurities have been cooked away) and Red Mountain iron ore. The resulting product was of high enough quality to compete with the metal being made in the North, and the successful experiment birthed a great city.

From No. 13, you can head back the way you came in to complete the short hike.

But if you're in the mood for more, head back but then turn left (east) and follow the Ike Maston Trail toward the Ishkooda No. 14 Mine. The trail is named for Ike Maston, who was a miner on the mountain from the late 1940s to the early 1960s and who is featured in the Red Mountain Oral History Project. He died in 2010.

The Ike Maston Trail ends as it intersects the No. 14 Mine Spur. Take a left and go up the mountain a short distance to find the portal of the No. 14 mine. A subsidence in the mountainside allows you a glimpse of the mine.

Head back down the No. 14 Mine Spur and take a diversion into an open area, where you'll find stone foundations of structures where ore was stored for loading onto the rail spur that served the area.

Now you can return by following the No. 14 Mine Spur to the BMRR South Trail and following it back to the main kiosk. Along the way, you can take a shortcut back by jumping on the Eureka Mines Trail. If you amble all the way back on BMRR South, remember to turn back left (east) when you intersect with the main line of that trail, following the signs to the parking lot.

Directions

See page 137.

REMNANTS OF IRON ORE–LOADING STRUCTURES LINE THE HILLSIDE ABOVE THE BIRMINGHAM MINERAL RAILROAD TRAIL. *(See Hike 16.)*

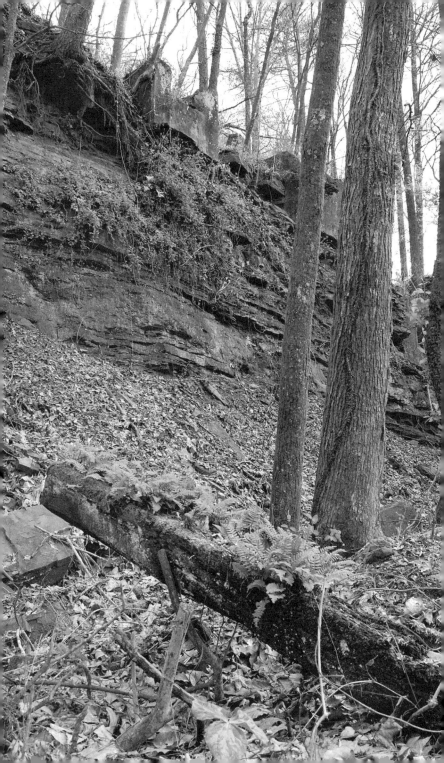

Ruffner Mountain Nature Preserve (Hikes 19–21)

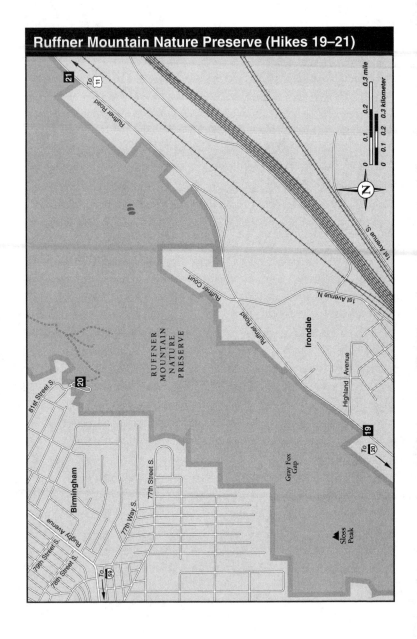

Ruffner Mountain
Nature Preserve

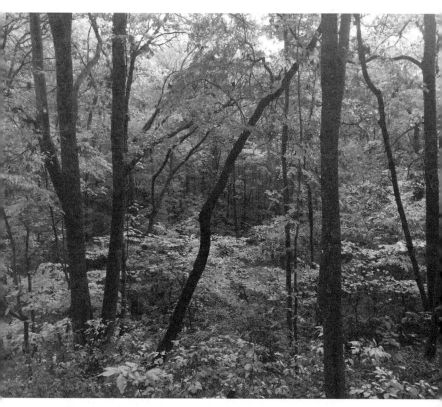

THE RIDGE & VALLEY TRAIL IS A GREAT SPOT FOR VIEWING COLORFUL FALL LEAVES. *(See Hike 19.)*

Ruffner Mountain Nature Preserve Overview

SITUATED ON A STRETCH OF RED MOUNTAIN that separates Irondale and Birmingham, Ruffner Mountain Nature Preserve is our "mother" nature park, our original walk in the woods within the city.

Minutes from downtown, you can be hiking through the hardwood forest out the spine of the mountain. Before long you're at the rocky overlook at Hawk's View, looking down at Jones Valley below: the planes landing and taking off from the airport, the city skyline in view. Up here, in the fresh air, you feel both far away from the city and right in it, all at the same time.

Ruffner Mountain is often the first place where kids look into the eyes of an owl, stroke a snake, or pet a bunny. The state's first nature-education center opened here back in the 1970s, and today the nonprofit that manages the preserve hosts a steady stream of school field trips, weekend programs, and summer camps.

Over the past decade, the preserve has been reborn. The nature center's campus now features a $15 million, LEED Gold–certified education and headquarters building as well an adjacent event pavilion. New trailheads and parking on the southeast side of the mountain provide access to an expanded trail system that now totals more than 12 miles, as well as new attractions. Eventually, Ruffner would also like to see restoration of and guest access to the 100-foot-tall fire tower atop the mountain, which would offer views rivaling Vulcan's.

From the late 1880s until 1953, Sloss Iron and Steel Company mined iron ore from this part of the mountain, sending it rolling by rail to Sloss Furnaces just east of downtown. Limestone was also quarried from the mountaintop, and you can still see the clear evidence of man's shifting and shaping of the land.

But after the mining ceased, the land was left alone to recover for decades. In the 1970s, an ill-conceived plan for an apartment complex on the mountain slope led neighbors to band together to stop it. In the end, the city of Birmingham ended up with possession of a chunk of wooded mountainside, and out of the opposition movement a nonprofit was formed to take care of the land and teach people about the value of nature.

Since that time, the park has grown to more than 1,000 acres, including 500 acres acquired by the state's Forever Wild program and 500 acres owned by the city of Birmingham.

Throughout its existence, Ruffner Mountain has emphasized its identity as a preserve. Don't expect zip lines. Don't bring your mountain bike (though polite trail runners are welcome). Leashed dogs are also welcome (just make sure to clean up after them).

And it's not all about solitude and communing with nature. Check the calendar for a regular series of events like Beer on the Back Porch (music, beverages, and dinner), Art on R Mountain, and native-plant sales.

Spring brings ephemeral wildflowers. Late in spring, the frog chorus gets loud around the wetlands area on the southeast side of the mountain. And in summer, you can escape the heat of the concrete with a shady walk out to the sunny quarries, where hardy purple asters and goldenrod color the limestone overlooks. Ruffner is a great place to catch the changing leaves in fall and to burn off a holiday meal in the winter.

Trailheads

You can access Ruffner's trails from three principal trailheads, each providing a slightly different experience.

The classic introduction is to start at Ruffner Mountain's **Tree House Visitor Center,** at the dead end of 81st Street South in Birmingham's South East Lake neighborhood. The eco-friendly Tree House is worth a visit in itself, but while you're there you can also see animals and other exhibits when the center is open. There are picnic and restroom facilities here, as well as access to most of the trails, including a system of short trails around the center and longer trails out to the quarry and overlooks.

On the southeastern side of the mountain, you can park at the **Irondale Ball Fields Trailhead** on Ruffner Road, where you can get on the Ridge & Valley Trail. Farther out Ruffner Road toward Trussville is the **Ruffner Road Trailhead,** which offers access to the Pipeline Trail and wetlands area.

Trails

All trails are color coded and well marked. The **Trillium Trail, Marian Harnach Nature Trail,** and **Geology Trail** are short trails near the visitor center. The Trillium Trail is a good place to look for spring wildflowers. The Geology Trail features Turtle Rock, a good spot for pre-K rock climbers.

The **Quarry Trail** is the main artery from the Tree House Visitor Center to the most scenic spots on the mountain. It's a nice hike for distance and isn't particularly steep since you start fairly close to the top of the mountain. The **Hollow Tree Trail** and **Silent Journey Trail** both branch off from and return to the Quarry Trail, offering a way to make the trip back a little different. When the Quarry Trail reaches an intersection called Gray Fox Gap, you have a choice. You can explore the quarries, take the **Overlook Trail** up for bird's-eye view of the quarry and the city beyond, or you can take **Possum Loop,** which provides extra distance and nice but less-dramatic city views.

The **Ridge & Valley Trail** is also accessible at Gray Fox Gap, but I recommend starting at the Irondale Ball Fields Trailhead. Ridge & Valley is rated as the most strenuous of the trails. It gains and loses elevation several times, tracing the contours of the southeast side of the mountain. If you're up for the challenge, it's worth it, especially in combination with the **Crusher Trail,** which branches off the Ridge & Valley Trail in a loop that shows off one of the best-preserved relics of mining operations: a huge ore crusher left out in the middle of the woods.

The **Pipeline Trail** begins at the Ruffner Road Trailhead and follows a gas pipeline. It's wide and flat, and if you look closely you'll notice that in places you are paralleling an old rail bed. The **Lizard Loop** branches off to the north, while taking the Pipeline Trail south gets you to the **Wetlands Trail,** with its adjacent picnic area, and the **Sandstone Ridge Trail.** The **Buckeye Trail** climbs the mountain and connects to the rest of the trail system.

More Information

DIRECTIONS: Ruffner can be a little tricky to find. The Tree House Visitor Center is at 1214 81st St. S., where 81st Street dead-ends. To get here, you can take Oporto-Madrid Boulevard, which runs from Montevallo Road in the Eastwood Mall area to I-59's Exit 131 in East Lake. From I-59, you head south and east on Oporto-Madrid toward Eastwood. After you cross Fifth Avenue South, take a left onto Rugby Avenue. Coming from Eastwood, you'll be headed north on Oporto-Madrid. After you pass 76th Street South, the road will curve to the left. Be looking for a right on Rugby Avenue. (There is often a sign to the center at this turn, though it's been known to disappear.) Follow Rugby to 81st Street and turn right up the mountain. Keep straight.

To get to the Ruffner Road trailheads in Irondale, you can take Georgia Road out of Woodlawn to its intersection with Ruffner Road and head left (northeast) on Ruffner, or take Montevallo Road or US 78 (Crestwood Boulevard) to 16th Street South in Irondale. Take 16th Street north toward the mountain and the Ruffner baseball and softball fields. When 16th Street intersects Ruffner Road, take a right, heading northeast.

The Irondale Ball Fields Trailhead is across the street from the baseball fields, where parking is allowed. Look for a Ruffner Mountain Nature Preserve sign.

The Ruffner Road Trailhead is farther north; look for auto-parts businesses on the right side of Ruffner Road, then look left for Ruffner Mountain Nature Preserve signs, a small gravel parking lot, and a gated entrance.

If you're coming from Trussville, Ruffner Road branches off US 11 (Gadsden Highway) south of I-459. From that direction, you'll come to the Ruffner Road Trailhead first and the Irondale Ball Fields Trailhead second.

ACCESS: The trails are open daily, sunrise–sunset; the Tree House Visitor Center is open Tuesday–Saturday, 9 a.m.–5 p.m., and Sunday, 1–5 p.m. If you arrive before the visitor center is open or plan to return to your car after the 5 p.m. closing time, park outside the gate on 81st Street South. The gate is locked when the center closes. Admission is free, but a $2-per-person donation would be appreciated. Or you can help support the preserve by becoming a member ($35 for individuals, $45 for families).

MAPS: An excellent digital park map is available at **ruffnermountain.org/visitors/trail -maps**. Or pick up a map at the visitor center. Remember, the visitor center is managed by a nonprofit. Donations are appreciated.

FACILITIES: The Tree House Visitor Center has restrooms, exhibits, and a small gift shop. The picnic pavilion and porch across from the center have restrooms, tables, and vending machines. The two trailheads on Ruffner Road have information kiosks, but don't count on getting a map there. The wetlands area has picnic tables, a picnic pavilion, and a portable toilet, and benches are sprinkled throughout the trail system.

WHEELCHAIR ACCESS: Varies; see individual hike profiles.

COMMENTS: Ruffner Mountain was mined and quarried. Stay on the trails. Watch out for steep cliffs and dropoffs. Keep an eye on your kids.

CONTACTS: 205-833-8264, **ruffnermountain.org**. For in-depth information on the geology and ecology of the mountain, visit **trekbirmingham.com/places/ruffner-mountain**. For more information about the wetlands area, including photos, visit **alabamabirdingtrails.com/sites /ruffner-mountain-wetlands.**

19 Ruffner Mountain Nature Preserve:
Ridge & Valley Loop

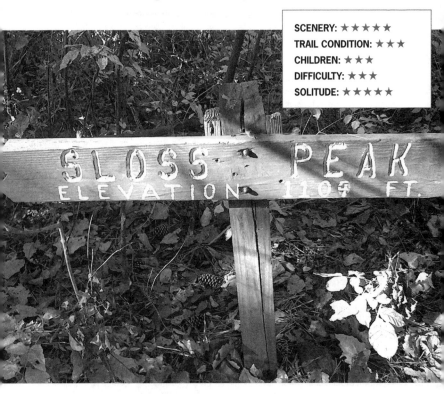

SCENERY: ★ ★ ★ ★ ★
TRAIL CONDITION: ★ ★ ★
CHILDREN: ★ ★ ★
DIFFICULTY: ★ ★ ★
SOLITUDE: ★ ★ ★ ★ ★

GPS TRAILHEAD COORDINATES: N33° 32.626' W86° 42.619'

DISTANCE & CONFIGURATION: 3.5-mile loop

HIKING TIME: 3 hours

HIGHLIGHTS: Great fall color; mountain-climb; mining ruins, including an enormous ore crusher; views of the city; views of the city from the mountaintop; a nice challenge with a lot of elevation gain

ELEVATION: 800' at trailhead, 1,104' at Sloss Peak

ACCESS, MAPS: See previous page.

FACILITIES: Benches

WHEELCHAIR ACCESS: None

COMMENTS: Watch for poison ivy—there's a lot of it.

Overview

For me, this was a great discovery: a quick, convenient, and vigorous getaway hike, with great fall color and interesting sights and scenery. It's challenging in that it gains and loses elevation as it proceeds up and down the draws on the southeast flank of the mountain before climbing to the ridgetop. The ore crusher is a must-see monument to Ruffner Mountain's mining past. This route also gives you access to the mountaintop quarry and city overlooks that are highlights of any visit to Ruffner Mountain.

Route Details

This hike begins at Ruffner's newest access point: a trailhead across the street from Irondale's community ballpark, on 16th Street South not far from the end of Montevallo Road. Hikers can park at the ball fields across the street from the trailhead.

The route follows the Ridge & Valley Trail along the flank of the mountain to its intersection with the Crusher Trail. It then follows the Crusher Trail on a scenic loop and, returning, continues the ascent to the top of the mountain and the Quarry Trail. Once on the Quarry Trail, you'll hike to the quarry and overlooks. When you're ready to return to your car, you can hike down a different section of the Ridge & Valley Trail, which branches off the Quarry Trail at Gray Fox Gap. That will take you down the mountain and back to the ball fields. It's a 3.5-mile hike that combines some challenge with beautiful scenery and varied terrain.

Follow the trail to the right (northeast) from the entrance, avoiding the TRAIL CLOSED sign that keeps you from going straight uphill. Shortly thereafter comes another split—follow the sign pointing right to Ridge & Valley Trail. The trail is marked with orange blazes.

Very quickly after you start the hike, you'll find yourself immersed in the forest, though I-20 still produces a background hum. I set out on an early morning. I looked up to see a hawk drop from his roost, gliding away from me, headed to breakfast. The leaves

Ruffner Mountain Nature Preserve: Ridge & Valley Loop

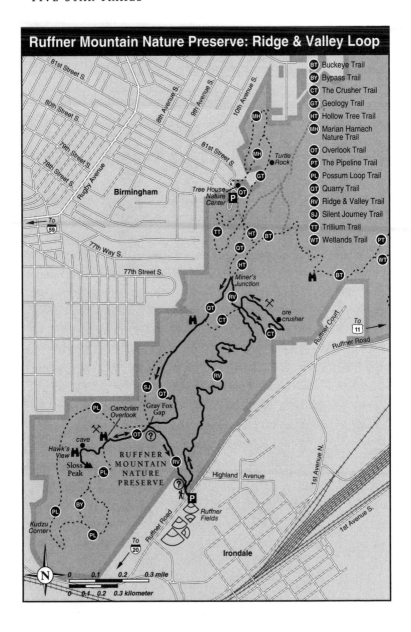

BT Buckeye Trail
BY Bypass Trail
CT The Crusher Trail
GT Geology Trail
HT Hollow Tree Trail
MH Marian Harnach Nature Trail
OT Overlook Trail
PT The Pipeline Trail
PL Possum Loop Trail
QT Quarry Trail
RV Ridge & Valley Trail
SJ Silent Journey Trail
TT Trillium Trail
WT Wetlands Trail

81st Street S.
80th Street S.
79th Street S.
78th Street S.
Rugby Avenue
8th Avenue S.
9th Avenue S.
10th Avenue S.
81st Street S.

Birmingham

To 59

77th Way S.
77th Street S.

Tree House Nature Center
Turtle Rock
Miner's Junction
ore crusher

Ruffner Court
To 11
Ruffner Road

Cambrian Overlook
Gray Fox Gap
cave
Hawk's View
Sloss Peak

RUFFNER MOUNTAIN NATURE PRESERVE

Kudzu Corner

Highland Avenue

1st Avenue N.

To 20
Ruffner Road
Ruffner Fields

Irondale

1st Avenue S.

N

0   0.1   0.2   0.3 mile
0   0.1   0.2   0.3 kilometer

were turning: sweet-gum red, hickory and tulip-poplar yellow. The tree trunks were dark, and the green of pine served as a backdrop.

Looking down, I found the earth was red, colored by the iron that made the mountain famous. Tree roots were colored in the same rusty tint. Other rocks near the dry stream bed were moss-covered green. I spent a good deal of time thinking about how the peak of fall colors should be a local holiday.

On this portion of the hike, you're traversing the contours of a succession of draws, each one offering a slightly different assembly of vegetation, each its own little kingdom. At the center of each is a creeklike corridor, where water drains from the slopes and escapes down the mountain, eventually collecting to form the headwaters of Shades Creek.

About 1.2 miles into the hike, you come to what appears to be a four-way intersection. Downhill, to the southeast, is the loop that leads to the iron ore crusher. Uphill is a connection to the mountaintop trail system.

Go see the crusher. It's a short, pretty walk down the draw to find it. The crusher is a huge, bulbous iron machine mounted on a stone foundation. Apparently, iron ore was loaded into it so it could be crushed into smaller chunks before it was transported to the furnaces downtown. Nowadays, downtown seems so far away from this remote spot shrouded in a jungle of privet.

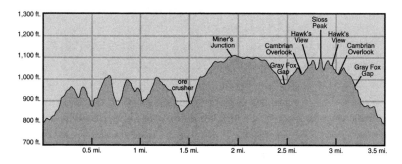

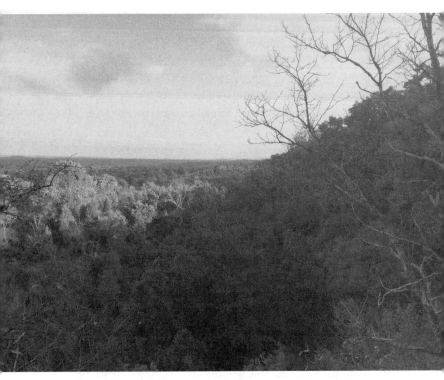

RUFFNER HAS SEVERAL SPOTS NEAR THE QUARRY WHERE YOU CAN TAKE IN WIDE PANORAMAS, LIKE THIS ONE FROM THE CAMBRIAN OVERLOOK.

Continue the loop back to the original intersection and then proceed to the right, following the orange blazes up the hill to complete the Ridge & Valley Trail's ascent of the mountain.

At the top of the ridge, at Miner's Junction, you'll intersect the Quarry Trail. Head toward the quarry, the opposite direction from the visitor center.

This is the main artery of the trail system at Ruffner, and it leads to the most scenic spots in the park. At Gray Fox Gap, take a look at the signs and get your bearings. You'll return to this spot and take the Ridge & Valley Trail back downhill to your car.

Having come this far and having gotten this close to the overlooks and the quarry, I couldn't resist pressing on. I provide more detail of the remaining stretch in the Hawk's View hike (see next page). Suffice it to say the routes that people take in this area are various. Sometimes it's hard to figure out where the real trail is. Don't worry too much about that, but do be careful not to fall off the cliffs overlooking the quarry and the high spots at Hawk's View. From Hawk's View, you can also follow the signs to Sloss Peak, a high point on the mountain, to complete your total elevation gain.

Whatever you've chosen to do, make your way back to Gray Fox Gap. From there, take the Ridge & Valley Trail downhill to the ball fields and your car.

Nearby Attractions

If you're in the area, you might want to start or end your hike with a visit to two landmark restaurants in Irondale. **Golden Rule Bar-B-Q** (205-956-2678, **goldenrulebbq.biz**) traces its roots back to 1891, with the opening of a roadside stop for travelers on the road to Atlanta. The original location, not far from the site of today's restaurant on US 78 (officially 2504 Crestwood Blvd.), served pork plates and beer and, after the invention of the automobile, occasionally did car repair.

The **Irondale Cafe,** a meat-and-three mecca in downtown Irondale (1906 First Ave. N.; 205-956-5258, **irondalecafe.com**), opened in 1928. The original restaurant was owned by Bess Fortenberry. Her niece, Fannie Flagg, set her novel *Fried Green Tomatoes at the Whistle Stop Cafe* in Whistle Stop, a fictional version of Irondale. The novel was made into a movie, *Fried Green Tomatoes,* and the restaurant is today a draw for fans of Southern cooking, the movie, and the trains that pass through downtown Irondale on a regular basis.

Directions

See page 163 for directions to the Irondale Ball Fields Trailhead.

20

Ruffner Mountain Nature Preserve:
Tree House to Hawk's View

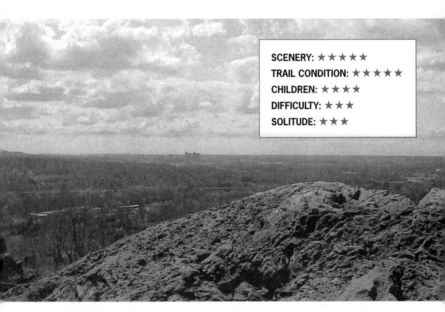

SCENERY: ★ ★ ★ ★ ★
TRAIL CONDITION: ★ ★ ★ ★ ★
CHILDREN: ★ ★ ★ ★
DIFFICULTY: ★ ★ ★
SOLITUDE: ★ ★ ★

GPS TRAILHEAD COORDINATES: N33° 33.569' W86° 42.386'

DISTANCE & CONFIGURATION: 3-mile out-and-back

HIKING TIME: 2.5 hours

HIGHLIGHTS: Tree House Visitor Center, ridgetop forest, wildflowers, fossil hunting and exploring in an old limestone quarry, and views of the city skyline from the rocky overlook at Hawk's View

ELEVATION: 850' at the beginning, 1,106' at the peak

ACCESS, MAPS, FACILITIES: See page 163.

WHEELCHAIR ACCESS: The visitor center is accessible.

COMMENTS: Stay on the trails, and look out for steep edges.

Overview

This is the classic urban-forest hike, offering a quick getaway from the city and an immediate immersion in the woods. It culminates in some scenic highlights that can't be beat. Because you start close to the mountaintop, there isn't a great deal of elevation change, so you get to stretch your legs without huffing and puffing. This route follows the Quarry Trail to its end, where you can connect to the Overlook Trail. You can even add on the Possum Loop to the end for a total distance of closer to 5 miles.

Route Details

This hike has a special place in my heart because it was the scene of my first successful date with the woman who would become my wife. Ivy was in Birmingham for a short time for a physical-therapy internship. She'd spent years out west after college, and she appreciated the outdoors. Ruffner proved to be a card well played.

I was letting her in on a beautiful secret. After a woodland walk, we sat on the rocks at Hawk's View, looking out at the wide valley far below. There was that little dizziness you feel at being at the edge of something. And indeed we were.

In the years since, we've returned often to Ruffner to introduce the kids and to enjoy new additions and improvements, but this classic hike remains a favorite.

Start at the Tree House Visitor Center. Aside from checking out the exhibits, appreciate the building itself, how it's built to live lightly on the land. Go out to the far end of its deck and see how it feels to be in the treetops.

When you're ready to head out, find the trailhead and follow the signs for the Quarry Trail. The initial path of the trail doesn't seem exactly right directionally. You end up crossing a paved road that leads back into the parking area. Walk straight across it and hit another information kiosk. From this second start, the trail conforms more to my sense of direction. Continue heading out the ridge, and continue to enjoy the plant-identification signs along the way.

You soon have the option of taking a spur, the Hollow Tree Trail, which is fine to take if you want some variety or a little more

Ruffner Mountain Nature Preserve: Tree House to Hawk's View

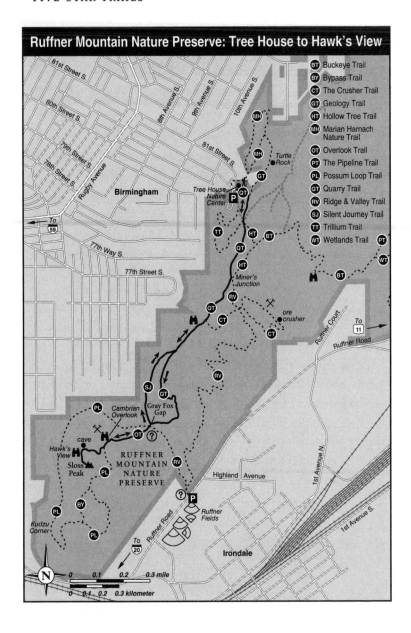

BT Buckeye Trail
BY Bypass Trail
CT The Crusher Trail
GT Geology Trail
HT Hollow Tree Trail
MH Marian Harnach Nature Trail
OT Overlook Trail
PT The Pipeline Trail
PL Possum Loop Trail
QT Quarry Trail
RV Ridge & Valley Trail
SJ Silent Journey Trail
TT Trillium Trail
WT Wetlands Trail

elevation change. It reconnects to the Quarry Trail a little farther down the ridge. However, the namesake Hollow Tree, a 150-year-old tulip poplar, is only a memory—it was damaged and had to be cut down. If you do take the Hollow Tree Trail, it mounts the ridge and then turns right, following a gravel access road up the mountain for a bit before descending back to the Quarry Trail.

I prefer the Quarry Trail. The trees along the trail, mostly tulip poplars and oaks, seem extraordinarily tall. More often than not, their tops are being tousled by the air currents moving up and down the mountain. Most look like they've spent most of their energy growing up rather than filling in wide, but some, particularly the tulip poplars, have tremendous girth as well.

There are a couple of diversions along the Quarry Trail worth seeing: a peaceful spot with a bench and a valley overlook, and an experimental longleaf-pine reforestation area. You also have the option of taking the Silent Journey Trail, which branches off and then parallels the Quarry Trail downhill from it, and then rejoins it. I recommend trying it on the way out or the way back. There are some nice rock formations along this trail.

Whichever way you go, you end up at Gray Fox Gap, where you're presented with several options. If you want a long walk, you can circle around on Possum Loop, a nice hike that ends up adding an

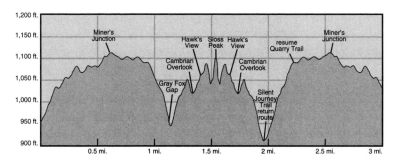

extra 2 miles to the adventure. It is a mostly level walk on an old road or roadbed and this part of the mountain. It's lightly traveled but in several spots offers nice city views. Plus you can find unexplained remains and ruins along the way.

Unless you're in a desperate hurry to get to Hawk's View, take a diversion into the limestone quarry. It's an unusual landscape—rocky, moonlike, sparsely vegetated. If you look closely at the rock, you can find the fossils of ocean creatures deposited here more than 488 million years ago, when the area was covered by a shallow sea. The limestone was quarried for use in removing impurities from the crushed and melted iron ore.

Retrace your steps and follow the signs to the overlook. You can choose from several paths. You get a nice overhead view of the quarry from the Cambrian Overlook, and you can see out to the surrounding country. Be very careful, however, near the edge of the quarry and at Hawk's View. It's a long way down. You should also look out for holes and pits in the limestone on the way up to Hawk's View.

If you look carefully, there's a small crevice and cave in limestone boulders on the way to Hawk's View. Visitors are discouraged from exploring caves on Ruffner property. This one doesn't go much of anywhere, but it does get dark and cramped quickly—not for claustrophobics. Passing that by, you arrive at a view of wide-open sky: Hawk's View. From this rocky precipice, you're looking out over Red Gap, where Red Mountain dips low, forming the corridor where I-20 and other transportation arteries pass through the mountain. Across Red Gap, Red Mountain rises again to form the ridge that supports Vulcan. The airport is below, to the north. The cluster of towers downtown is visible to the west. There is enough room to sit down against the rocks here.

If you've never seen Hawk's View, it will give you a new perspective on Birmingham. It's certainly worth the hike.

Directions

See page 163 for directions to the visitor center.

21

Ruffner Mountain
Nature Preserve:
Wetlands Retreat

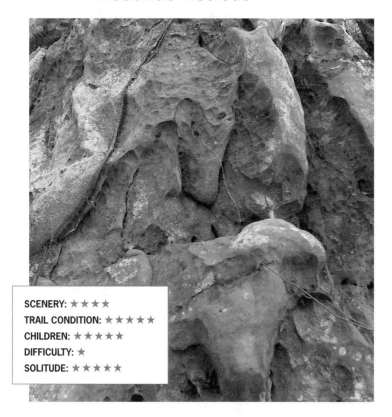

SCENERY: ★ ★ ★ ★
TRAIL CONDITION: ★ ★ ★ ★ ★
CHILDREN: ★ ★ ★ ★ ★
DIFFICULTY: ★
SOLITUDE: ★ ★ ★ ★ ★

GPS TRAILHEAD COORDINATES: N33° 33.522' W86° 41.339'

DISTANCE & CONFIGURATION: 2-mile out-and-back with 2 small balloons

HIKING TIME: 2 hours

HIGHLIGHTS: Easy walk to a spring-fed waterside retreat and picnic area, with a short side trip available to a rock formation for climbing. Spring and summer wildflowers.

ELEVATION: 777' at the trailhead, rising to 857'

ACCESS, MAPS, FACILITIES: See page 163.

WHEELCHAIR ACCESS: Gravel road to wetlands

COMMENTS: You may hear gunfire in this area, and a lot of it. Fear not—it's a nearby shooting range.

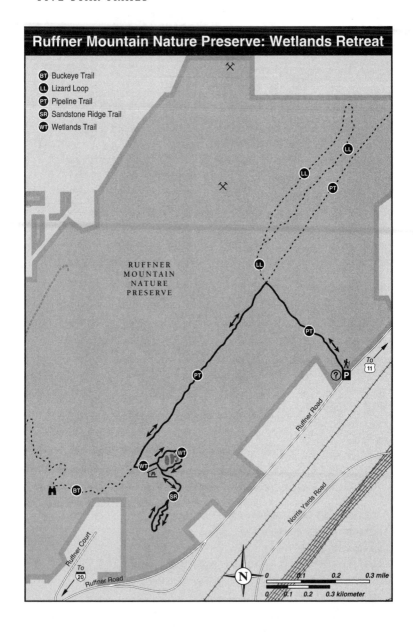

Ruffner Mountain Nature Preserve: Wetlands Retreat

- **BT** Buckeye Trail
- **LL** Lizard Loop
- **PT** Pipeline Trail
- **SR** Sandstone Ridge Trail
- **WT** Wetlands Trail

RUFFNER
MOUNTAIN
NATURE
PRESERVE

Overview

A wide, level path to a spring-fed wetlands with boardwalk and picnic facilities. Frogs croak among the irises and cattails. Birds abound. An easy side hike leads to a small ridge of unusual sandstone boulders—remnants of a prehistoric seashore—perfect for junior explorers.

Route Details

This may be one of the most idyllic spots you can find for a picnic, especially if you have children in tow. It's a relatively short walk over level ground to the wetlands, where any trip around the boardwalk is guaranteed to set off leaping frogs. Kids can play on boulders on the banks of the wetlands; for more adventure, it's a short walk to a sandstone outcropping that offers more climbing.

For this hike, we take advantage of the northernmost Ruffner Road entrance to the nature preserve and enter at that gate, which is also an access road for a natural-gas pipeline. Walk in from the road 0.3 mile and intersect the gas pipeline. If you want to throw in a little extra walking, the Lizard Loop lies straight across the pipeline. The loop is a mile long and, for the most part, follows what was once a rail bed.

To proceed to the wetlands, take a left, to the southwest. You'll soon see a facility related to the gas pipeline; steer clear and proceed

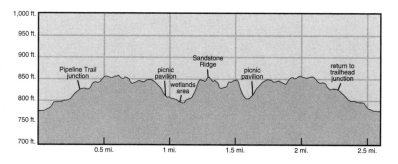

past it. As you walk along this stretch, look off into the woods toward the mountainside for evidence of an old elevated rail bed. In several places, you can still see stone culverts built to allow water running off the mountain to pass under and through the rail embankment. This was part of the Birmingham Mineral Railroad, also known as the L&N, a railroad loop that allowed trains to be loaded with iron ore from the mines on Red Mountain, and from there to move down into Jones Valley and the furnaces from Bessemer to Birmingham. Portions of this railroad have been turned into the Vulcan Trail and some of the hiking trails at Red Mountain Park.

The pipeline road is gravel, which means this isn't a deep-woods walk, but it also means that the adjacent land gets plenty of sunlight, allowing for thriving patches of wildflowers.

A little less than a mile into the walk, you reach a junction. If you were to continue straight, you could pick up the Buckeye Trail, climb the mountain, and connect with the other trails in the system. From this spot, the visitor center is about 1 steep mile away.

Instead, take a left, following the signs to the wetlands. You'll first pass through a wide meadow. To your right you'll notice a large picnic pavilion. Closer to the wetlands are additional picnic tables in the shade, as well as a collection of boulders for sitting and climbing. As I was approaching, a bluebird flashed against the green, darting and swooping, then came to rest on a tree branch above the picnic area. This appearance of good fortune made me stop and notice how many distinct bird songs I could hear. I can't give you a numerical answer; I'll just say a lot. There's nothing like a little break in the trees and a little water supply to draw them in droves.

The wetlands themselves are a series of small ponds and marshes that you can walk in and through along a raised wooden boardwalk. At the right time of year and the right time of day, you'll hear frogs singing along with the birds, and if you don't hear them croaking and chirping, you'll hear them jumping as you walk along and they evacuate their pond-side perches among the cattails. On the northern bank of the wetlands, you can see the springs that gurgle up to feed the wetlands. These waters eventually find their way to form the headwaters of Shades Creek, and thus you'll also see them at the Irondale Furnace in Mountain Brook, in Jemison Park, and then later along the Shades Creek Greenway.

In the picnic area, you'll see signs for a trail leading off into the woods to Sandstone Ridge. Geologists say this rock outcropping is part of the Hartselle Sandstone, deposits of sand from a barrier-island system when the area was seaside real estate 330 million years ago. You can see hints of that ancient sandy beach in tiny sparkling quartz crystals embedded in a line of boulders, some as tall as 10 feet, which pop up out of the woods. Erosion has sculpted the boulders into dripping patterns that call to mind a wave- and wind-washed sandcastle. The trail loops through, with one side tracing the low side, where the wear patterns and oakleaf hydrangeas make for a nice walk, and the upper side, where the sparkling rock and the little glimpse of mountains are a treat. All along the way, they're the right scale for miniature mountain-climbing expeditions. Once upon a time, this sandstone deposit was mined and used by the nearby Pioneer Glass-works to make glass.

Nearby Attractions

See Nearby Attractions for the Ridge & Valley Loop, page 169.

Directions

See page 163 for directions to the northernmost trailhead on Ruff-ner Road.

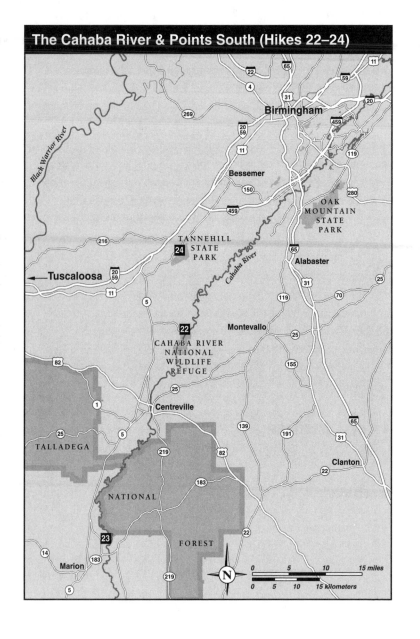

The Cahaba River & Points South (Hikes 22–24)

The Cahaba River & Points South

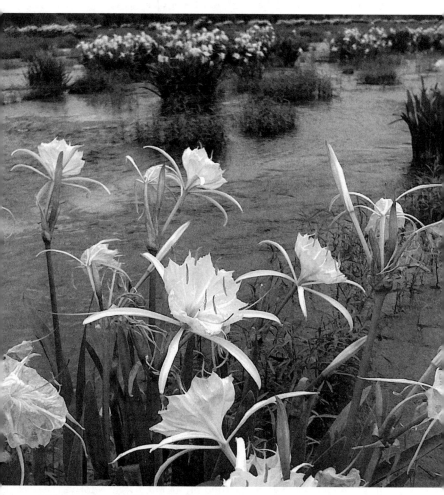

CAHABA LILIES BLOOM FROM ABOUT MOTHER'S DAY TO FATHER'S DAY IN THE CAHABA RIVER NATIONAL WILDLIFE REFUGE. *(See Hike 22.)*

Cahaba River & Points South Overview

THE HIKES IN THIS SECTION are along the Cahaba River basin south of Birmingham. The Cahaba has long been valued as a drinking-water resource. People living close to the river and a certain subset of folks in the know have always sought it out for its beauty and recreational value.

But only in the past couple of decades have people begun to appreciate what a truly special river it is. We knew it had those glorious, spring-blooming Cahaba lilies growing on its southern shoals. But few appreciated that it supported such a diversity of fish species, mussels, snails, crawfish, and turtles. Few waterways outside the tropics can compare.

The hikes in this section offer an introduction to the river at places with public access. The **Cahaba River National Wildlife Refuge** and **Perry Lakes Park** afford convenient river access. **Tannehill Ironworks Historical State Park,** also covered in this section, is connected to the Cahaba in that the pioneering ironworking operation made use of Cahaba feeder creeks to help drive production.

If these hikes whet your appetite, the **Cahaba River Society** (205-322-5326, **cahabariversociety.org**) is a good place to find more information. It has been working since 1988 to protect the river and deepen people's love for and appreciation of it. The society offers a regular schedule of guided paddles from spring to fall and is a key partner in the Cahaba Blueway Project, an effort to create a well-cataloged and consistently connected network of river access points from the headwaters all the way down to the river's merger with the Alabama River south of Selma.

And if you get down as far as Perry Lakes Park, you're on the edge of Alabama's Black Belt, once a region of cotton plantations. A nice synopsis of what you can find in Marion, Greensboro, and the surrounding area can be found at the **Alabama Tourism and Travel** website: **tinyurl.com/bamaroadtrip30.**

22 # Cahaba River National Wildlife Refuge

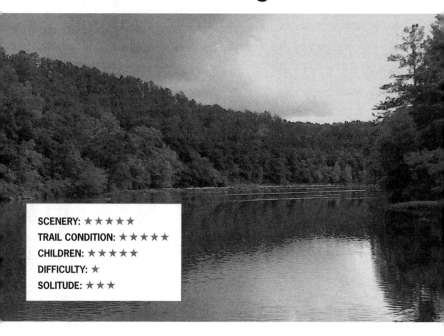

SCENERY: ★ ★ ★ ★ ★
TRAIL CONDITION: ★ ★ ★ ★ ★
CHILDREN: ★ ★ ★ ★ ★
DIFFICULTY: ★
SOLITUDE: ★ ★ ★

GPS TRAILHEAD COORDINATES: N33° 05.689' W87° 03.426'

DISTANCE & CONFIGURATION: 3-mile out-and-back

HIKING TIME: 2 hours (including time for lily-gazing)

HIGHLIGHTS: The Cahaba River; the world's largest known concentration of Cahaba lilies; swimming; fishing

ELEVATION: 346' at the start, 271' at the turnaround

ACCESS: Outdoor facilities open daily, sunrise–sunset; no fees

MAPS: Available at **fws.gov/cahabariver;** brochures available at kiosk; USGS *West Blocton East Quadrangle*

FACILITIES: None

WHEELCHAIR ACCESS: None

COMMENTS: Rain upstream can cause the river to rise and the lilies to be submerged. If you choose to wade or swim, you need shoes and should watch out for slick rocks and isolated swift currents.

CONTACTS: Refuge manager, 256-848-7085, **cahabariver@fws.gov; fws.gov/cahabariver** or **cahabariversociety.org** for additional resources.

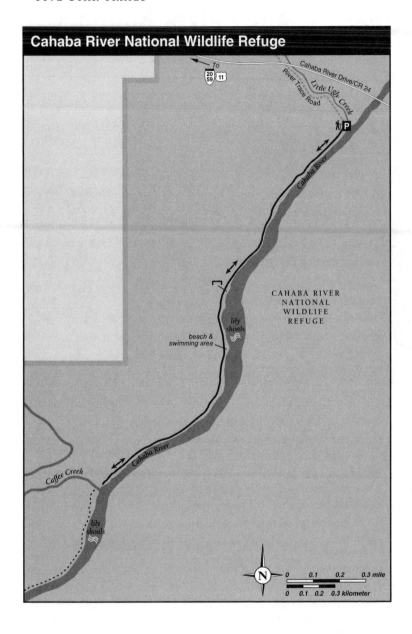

Cahaba River National Wildlife Refuge

To
20 59 11

Cahaba River Drive/CR 24

Little Ugly Creek

River Trace Road

🚶 🅿

Cahaba River

CAHABA RIVER
NATIONAL
WILDLIFE
REFUGE

lily shoals

beach & swimming area

Cahaba River

Caffee Creek

lily shoals

N

0   0.1   0.2   0.3 mile

0   0.1   0.2   0.3 kilometer

Overview

This riverside hike in the Cahaba River National Wildlife Refuge gives you access to canoe launches, swimming holes, fishing spots, and great views of the river. Between Mother's Day and Father's Day each year, it is the spot of one of Alabama's scenic wonders: the blooming of the world's largest known concentration of shoals lilies, known locally as Cahaba lilies.

Route Details

This hike follows a riverside gravel road from where it meets the river in the wildlife refuge to where the road dead-ends at Caffee Creek. Then you walk back.

You can't get lost or veer off the trail. You can shorten it by driving the gravel road straight to the lilies. You can even float this hike. Launch a canoe at the beginning, float downstream, and hike back up to your car from Caffee Creek.

However you choose to do it, it's well worth the effort.

The 3,500-acre Cahaba River National Wildlife Refuge in Bibb County protects a 3-mile stretch of one of North America's most biodiverse rivers.

From its headwaters in the mountains north and east of Birmingham, the Cahaba River trickles from mountain springs, tumbles through rocky rapids, and snakes through subdivisions. Its waters are siphoned off to provide Birmingham with its largest single source of drinking water. Along its course, the Cahaba receives the runoff from all the roads and parking lots in the watershed south of Red Mountain. The residue of what we put on our yards and the trash we toss in the street eventually returns in tubes, pipes, and culverts to the river. What's flushed down our household drains is treated and returned to the river.

Despite the punches it takes from us, the river to the south still manages to support a tremendous variety of aquatic life. Cahaba lilies, those rare and glorious white flowers, are found more abundantly here than anywhere else on Earth. The river supports 69 rare and imperiled species, including 10 fish and freshwater mussel species listed under the Endangered Species Act. There are more fish species per mile in the Cahaba than in any other similarly sized river in North America.

The word *Cahaba* is believed to be derived from Choctaw words meaning "water above" or "the river above." The refuge serves as a sanctuary for the celebration of the life-giving river, a pilgrimage spot, particularly during those high holy days in May and June when the lilies bloom.

If you want to visit when there's a crowd, try the **Cahaba River Ramble,** the annual early-May trail run hosted by the Cahaba River Society. Or later in May, you can catch the **Cahaba Lily Festival,** hosted by the nearby town of West Blocton.

I took my children the first weekend in June, a time when you can catch both the blooming lilies in the river's shoals and the blooming of the oakleaf hydrangeas, black-eyed Susans, and other wildflowers along the trail. We enjoyed sharing the refuge at this time of year with a good representation of fellow visitors, who came to swim, canoe, hike, and fish.

We parked at the pullout on River Trace Road, where the road first reaches the river (there is a canoe launch there). We proceeded downstream along the gravel road, which is shaded by a dense canopy of hardwoods. The river travels a narrow valley here, and if you look to the ridges on either side, you'll see that pine predominates in the uplands. Currently this is mostly loblolly pine, which timber companies planted to replace the original longleaf pine after earlier rounds of logging and mining. As part of an effort to restore the pine forest to its pre-industrial state, the U.S. Fish & Wildlife Service, which manages the refuge, is gradually reintroducing longleaf in the area.

Speaking of mining, look at a topographic map and you'll notice the sites of vanished mining towns and the names and designations of several coal mines, including the Piper and Hargrove Mines on refuge property. However, unless you know what you're looking for or you read some of the interpretive material, you probably won't detect evidence of it.

After a heavy rain, you will see contemporary pollution: the flotsam and jetsam of urban life carried downstream—everything from basketballs to plastic bottles, riding a chocolate torrent of sediment-laden water. But on our visit, the river was clear and relatively untroubled.

Not long after beginning the hike, you'll see the first of several rope swings that might tempt you. We checked the water depth under these attractions, and I'd strongly advise against trying them.

From the launch to the main beach and shoal of lilies, it's about a 1-mile walk. Along the way, you're tempted and teased with glimpses of the full glory of the river and the lilies. Boy Scouts have built benches for stopping along the way for quiet contemplation. Watch for the poison ivy that has crept up around some of them.

Arriving at the central sandy beach downstream from the largest shoal, you'll be overwhelmed looking back upstream and taking in what appears to be a football field's worth of green lilies topped with tall white blooms. The blooms seem to be faces turned skyward singing for joy.

If you're an early riser, consider coming out around dawn and watching the lilies emerge from the mist that is summoned by the rising sun from surface of the water. It feels like creation day, over and over. And on those early mornings, a tall wading heron may be your only companion.

If you choose to walk out into the shoals, note that the rocks can be slick, the underwater terrain uneven, and the current swift in spots. The rocks are crawling with aquatic snails. Along with the mussels found in the river, these humble creatures help clean and purify the water. Treat them with kindness.

There is some relatively deep protected water at the foot of the shoals where the sandy beach provides easy access. It's a nice place to swim, but bear in mind that there are currents here, especially if the water is high.

For a more secluded encounter with the river, you can continue down the river road. Lovely rock formations in the river punctuate the walk, and there's another smaller beach area where Caffee Creek meets the Cahaba.

This intersection marks the end of road and the end of the hike, though if you ford Caffee Creek, you can continue on a footpath farther downstream to where another large shoal of lilies awaits.

Nearby Attractions

The refuge was founded in 2002, and additional trails in the area are being developed. If you return to the paved road (Cahaba River Drive, or Bibb County Road 24), turn right, and cross the river, you'll come to a second parking lot, which provides access to the **Piper Trail,** a 1-mile trail on the ridge above the river. It ends at a platform overlooking the lily shoals.

Trails are also nearby at **Coke Ovens Park,** in West Blocton. This additional stop on the way to the refuge or on the way back will help you grasp the coal-mining history of the area. It's 3 miles west of the refuge on CR 24. For more information, go to **cokeovenspark.com.**

Directions

From I-20/I-59 toward Tuscaloosa, take Exit 97 (West Blocton/Centreville), turn south onto AL 5, and proceed south on US 11/AL 5. In about 3 miles, AL 5 branches off to the south at Woodstock.

Turn left onto AL 5 and travel about 7 miles, passing the turn to West Blocton. Signs at the next major intersection clearly point to the West Blocton bypass, also known as CR 24 or Cahaba River Drive. Continue 7 miles. Look for the refuge sign on the right—not the first wooden sign, which is a sign for the wildlife-management area, but the second sign. Shortly after the sign is a dirt road on the right, River Trace Road, which leads directly into the refuge. A kiosk at this entrance provides maps and information. Drive River Trace Road until you reach the river. There is pullout parking next to the canoe launch.

Perry Lakes Park & Barton's Beach

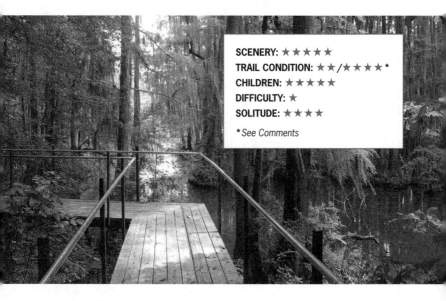

SCENERY: ★ ★ ★ ★ ★
TRAIL CONDITION: ★ ★ / ★ ★ ★ ★ ★ *
CHILDREN: ★ ★ ★ ★ ★
DIFFICULTY: ★
SOLITUDE: ★ ★ ★

See Comments

GPS TRAILHEAD COORDINATES: N32° 41.702' W87° 14.621'

DISTANCE & CONFIGURATION: 3-mile loop

HIKING TIME: The hike could be completed in an hour and a half, but plan to spend 3 hours to take in the sights, climb the tower, and maybe take a swim.

HIGHLIGHTS: Wander the shores of a cypress swamp. Climb a restored fire tower 100 feet to a perch in the canopy of Spanish moss–draped trees. Swim from a sandy beach on the Cahaba River. Enjoy an unexpected conglomeration of modern architecture built by students from Auburn University's Rural Studio.

ELEVATION: 154' at trailhead, with very little change throughout the hike

ACCESS: Daily, sunrise–sunset

MAPS: A roadside box offers maps, but it was empty when we visited. A rendering of the trail system is available at the website below.

FACILITIES: Bathrooms, running water, picnic tables, and a large pavilion. You might want to bring your own toilet paper, though.

WHEELCHAIR ACCESS: The roads and trails are unpaved, but to the extent that your chair can navigate gravel, there are sights worth seeing.

COMMENTS: The markings on the Devil's Walking Stick Trail were hard to follow when we visited, and the trail didn't seem to be frequently traveled. The trail to the birding tower, around the oxbow lakes, and out-and-back to the river is more well worn and scenic.

CONTACT: Perry Lakes Park, **perrylakes.org**

Perry Lakes Park & Barton's Beach

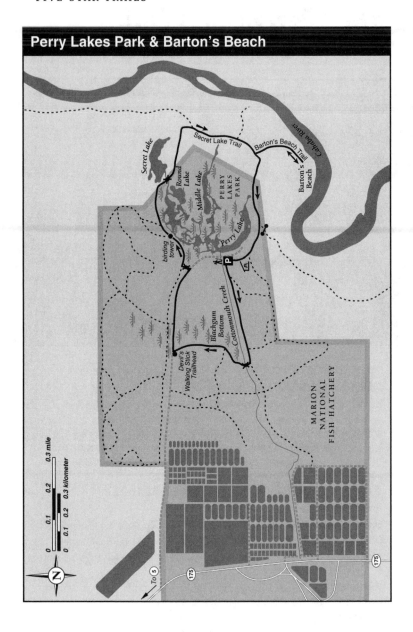

Overview

This loop hike, which can add up to about 3 miles of walking, is three hikes joined together. First, a woodland walk follows the Eagle Trail and Devil's Walking Stick Trail through old-growth forest with unusual tree and plant species. A second segment heads into the swamp toward Secret Lake and a 100-foot-tall former fire tower repurposed as a tree-canopy observation deck. Rejoining the road, a final diversion out to the river takes you to Barton's Beach for a swim. Put them together and you have the makings of a great day.

Route Details

Perry Lakes Park is one of the most unusual and wonderful spots I know. Part of its charm is what it is not. It's not a developed state park. It's not paved or manicured or bustling with visitors and staff. The amenities and trails developed here are a testament to community spirit and hard, unselfish work by an unusually broad array of folks.

The central natural features of the 600-acre park property are four oxbow lakes: pieces of what used to be river channel that were cut off when, more than 100 years ago, the Cahaba River changed course. Out of the waters of these low-lying remnants of river grew thickets of cypress and tupelo. Those trees, with their wide-based trunks, look as if they're swollen with the swamp water from which they rise. Their limbs hang thick with Spanish moss. Together they create patterns of shadows and reflections on the amber waters. Out there among the lily pads, you hear the occasional splash of fish, beaver, snake, or maybe alligator. The secluded forest draws a wide variety of birds, including bald eagles, which have nested nearby. And you can get a bird's-eye view of all this from a tower that takes you into the treetops.

The surrounding woodlands contain 60 species of native trees, and on our visit we saw plenty of wildlife: a hawk; a creekside full of bounding frogs; a fat cottonmouth snake swimming in the creek; and spiders, grasshoppers, and butterflies, including the painted lady and spicebush swallowtail.

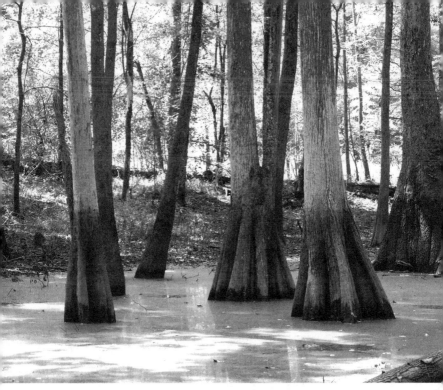

**THE SWOLLEN TRUNKS OF TUPELO AND CYPRESS TREES IN
BLACKGUM BOTTOM, ALONG THE DEVIL'S WALKING STICK TRAIL**

After you explore the swamp, you find yourself at 125-acre Barton's Beach, the largest sand-and-gravel bar on the Cahaba River. Preserved by The Nature Conservancy, this bar is a nesting ground for turtles. It's also a nice spot to sun and splash in the river and watch butterflies flutter. As the river rolls by, you can ponder the fact that this stretch of river is home to rare and wonderfully named fish like the skygazer shiner, crystal darter, and frecklebelly madtom. Also found under the water's surface are more than two dozen kinds of mussels, including species of conservational concern: the Alabama orb, heelsplitter, hickorynut, and ridged mapleleaf.

The nature is diverse here, and so is the cast of people and groups that make this park possible. Partners include Perry County; the city of Marion; and students and faculty from Judson College, Auburn University, Samford University, and the University of Alabama. The state of Alabama has reopened the fish hatchery that you'll see on the entrance road to the park, repurposed as the Alabama Center for Aquatic Biodiversity. Researchers at the center cultivate aquatic mussels and snails for reintroduction. These humble species were long ignored, and many were driven to extinction, but it turns out they are cornerstones of river ecology and water quality.

Let's get to our visit. Arriving at Perry Lakes Park, you'll immediately be struck by a collection of large structures that are a curious mix of weathered wood and spaceship-shiny steel. These landed here thanks to the astounding work of Auburn's architectural-education outpost in nearby Newbern, the Rural Studio. The first three buildings adjacent to the parking lot are the most avant-garde outhouses you've ever seen, complete with plumbing and contemplative views of nature. Nearby is a spacious picnic pavilion with the same spaceship chic. Students in the Rural Studio program also designed, built, and assembled a tin-roofed swinging bridge that leads out to the park's pièce de résistance: the restored fire tower that overlooks the swamp.

Instead of heading straight for that central attraction, we left the parking lot on the Eagle Trail, which follows a grassy, wide-open fire lane. I saw a hawk reeling in the sky, and the kids dawdled catching huge grasshoppers that we found in abundance. A little less than half a mile up this trail, we took a right across a narrow wooden bridge crossing Cottonmouth Creek.

As we crossed the bridge, the stream banks came alive with the hopping of frogs fleeing our approach. With all that jumping and movement, I was slightly nervous about crossing Cottonmouth Creek, especially after my son James reminded me that cottonmouth snakes love to eat frogs.

Safely on the other side, we found ourselves in a pawpaw patch. In the fall, pawpaw trees bear the largest edible fruit native to the United States. It's said to taste like a cross between a mango and a banana.

On the other side of the creek, follow a trail marked by square red-and-green metal signs with directional arrows. This becomes the Devil's Walking Stick Trail. Its highlights include an up-close look at a mini-swamp, Blackgum Bottom, where a collection of fat-trunked cypress and tupelo trees grow. At its end, the Devil's Walking Stick Trail connects to the entrance road.

Take a right, heading east, back toward the parking lot. A short distance later, about 1 mile into the hike, you'll see a bench at the roadside and signs pointing toward Secret Lake and the birding tower. Here, you'll cross a Rural Studio–constructed bridge over a creek. The trail to the tower and beyond follows high ground through a lovely maze of cypress and tupelo trees whose branches hang with Spanish moss.

The tower itself is a wonder, relocated from Atmore, Alabama. In 2005, Rural Studio students restored it and added safety enhancements. Reaching the top, you can survey the swamp, tree canopy, and surrounding hills.

As you continue deeper into the swamp, several benches offer solitude. After skirting Secret Lake, the trail veers to the right (southeast) and toward the river through a dense stand of privet, then emerges in a native grass meadow. It then connects with the entrance road. Taking a left, toward the south, you're shortly at Barton's Beach, a large sand-and-gravel bar on the Cahaba. It's a nice place to sun or soak. When we were there in late summer, it was also swarming with butterflies.

To return to your car, retrace your steps and follow the road back to the parking area. It's about a half-mile walk.

Directions

From I-20/I-59, take Exit 97 (Woodstock/West Blocton) and head south on US 11/AL 5. After 3.2 miles, take a left at Woodstock and head south on AL 5. After 35.8 miles, take a left on AL 175. Travel south 3.1 miles and look for the turn on the left to Perry Lakes Park and Barton's Beach. The Alabama Center for Aquatic Biodiversity is located at that intersection—if you drive past it, you've missed the turn.

24

Tannehill Ironworks Historical State Park

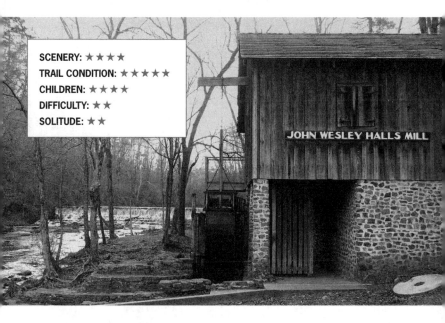

SCENERY: ★ ★ ★ ★
TRAIL CONDITION: ★ ★ ★ ★ ★
CHILDREN: ★ ★ ★ ★
DIFFICULTY: ★ ★
SOLITUDE: ★ ★

JOHN WESLEY HALLS MILL

GPS TRAILHEAD COORDINATES: N33° 14.980' W87° 04.267'

DISTANCE & CONFIGURATION: 5.5-mile balloon loop

HIKING TIME: 2.5 hours

HIGHLIGHTS: A restored 30-foot-tall Civil War–era furnace; a transplanted pioneer village; a great museum on the history of iron and industry; miles of hiking trails along historic routes on the 1,500-acre property; new mountain biking trails for exploring

ELEVATION: 450' at the museum, 600' at the peak of the hike

ACCESS: Daily, sunrise–sunset; admission to the park is $3 for adults, $1 for children. Museum hours are Monday–Friday, 8:30 a.m.–4:30 p.m.; Saturday, 9 a.m.–4:30 p.m.; and Sunday, 12:30–4:30 p.m. Admission is $2 for adults, $1 for children.

MAPS: Available at the camp store and the website below

FACILITIES: Restrooms, playground, store, picnic areas

WHEELCHAIR ACCESS: The museum and trails in the central grounds are accessible.

COMMENTS: If you want to make a weekend of it, there are rental cabins and camping options. Bring a bike and ride the new system of mountain bike trails. Check the calendar of events before you go—the park hosts events throughout the year, from trade days to music festivals to a haunted forest at Halloween.

CONTACT: 205-477-5711, **tannehill.org**

Tannehill Ironworks Historical State Park

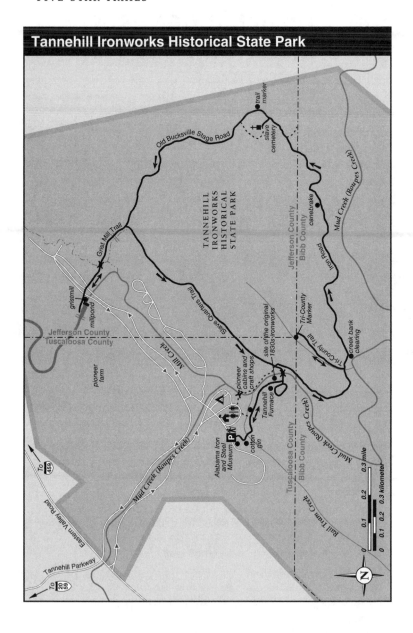

Overview

With its mix of history and nature, Tannehill is a great place for a quick getaway. This loop begins at the Alabama Museum of Iron and Steel and proceeds to the historic furnace site. It then wanders the woods along historic pathways, with stops at the intersection of three counties, a slave cemetery, and a replica of a 19th-century gristmill.

Route Details

Some weekends you really can still hear the blacksmith's hammer ringing at Tannehill Ironworks Historical State Park, the birthplace of the iron-and-steel industry in Greater Birmingham.

The centerpiece of the park is a massive restored furnace where pig iron was produced for the Confederacy until Union soldiers swept through and destroyed it in 1865. Earlier ironworking history on the site traces back to the 1830s. The park also hosts a collection of 19th-century buildings, from cabins to cotton gins, brought here from all over central Alabama.

In describing this hike, I'm describing what should probably be two separate visits: a historical exploration and a recreational wander through the woods. If you really want to digest the history, you could spend days here.

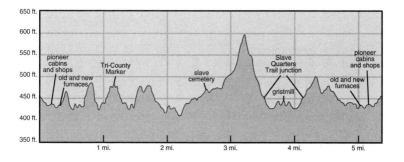

This hike begins and ends at the museum, where a visit is worth way more than the $2 admission charge. Even before you enter the doors, its displays on the geology and history of the site provide a valuable lay of the land. Tannehill lies at the rump end of the Appalachian Mountains, in a little pocket formed where Red Mountain and Shades Mountain come together and come to an end.

In the area are surface deposits of the iron ore for which Red Mountain is famous. That ore, plus deposits of limestone and a collection of creeks, made the area prime for iron manufacturing. Inside the museum, a timeline traces humans' use of iron and the development of the local industry. There's also an explanation of the basic extraction and production process, along with displays on Alabama's action in the Civil War and Tannehill's role in it.

In the last two years of the war, 70% of Confederate munitions came from the state's 13 operating blast furnaces, which included furnaces at Tannehill, the Oxmoor Furnace on Shades Creek near Red Mountain Park, and, farther up the creek, the "Old Cannonball Factory" in Mountain Brook. At its peak, Tannehill's battery of three blast furnaces could produce up to 22 tons of iron a day, most of it shipped to the Confederate arsenal at Selma.

In the spring of 1865, Union forces swept through Alabama and destroyed all but one of the functioning furnaces in the state. Tannehill was never successfully resurrected as a production site.

It was an abandoned ruin until the late 1960s and early 1970s, when a dedicated collection of local civic groups and preservationists banded together to save it and got it designated as a state historical park. The restoration efforts climaxed in 1976, when the furnaces were refired and iron was produced here one more time for a crowd of 10,000.

If you want to brush up on the history of Tannehill before you go, consult the online Encyclopedia of Alabama's entry. It was written by one of those preservationists who was key to the creation of the park: Jim Bennett, who went on to be elected Alabama's secretary of state.

After visiting the museum, find the trail to the furnace at the rear of the building. After descending a flight of stairs, the trail crosses the creek, then splits. I stuck to the low road, which proceeds behind the pioneer cabins, which are used by craftsmen and artists and are open on weekends between March and November.

Beyond the cabins, the trail parallels the creek that helped power the furnace. A waterwheel operated the bellows that pushed air into the furnace.

The furnace is a site to behold: an enormous 30-foot-tall chimney with arched openings at the base. It's amazing to think of the huge sandstone blocks being cut from nearby mountainsides and moved here by a labor force of slaves, without the aid of modern machinery. The area also includes an excavation of the original 1830s iron bloomery.

After exploring, cross the creek, called either Roupes or Mudd Creek, and follow the signs to the Iron Road, which heads off to the right, following the creek downstream. Throughout the rest of the hike, you will notice hike-and-bike trails connecting and diverging from the main hiking trail. This is a relatively new system of trails created by Birmingham Urban Mountain Pedalers. On this visit, we'll stay on the well-marked and well-mapped walking trails.

The Iron Road, the route used to move iron from the furnaces to the nearest stagecoach road, hugs a ridge above the creek, then turns and heads back into the woods. About half a mile from the furnace, you'll see the Tri-County Trail branching to the left, following a small creek up a draw.

I couldn't resist the chance to stand in three counties at one time, so I took the diversion. An engraved granite marker notes the intersection of Jefferson, Tuscaloosa, and Bibb Counties.

Returning to the main trail, you catch sight of Roupes Creek and can walk out to the bank here.

The Iron Road continues through moist bottomland forest for about a mile before reaching a side trail to the left that leads to the slave cemetery. When I visited, this spur was poorly marked. If you miss it, a better-marked path to the cemetery heads off from the Old Bucksville Stage Road.

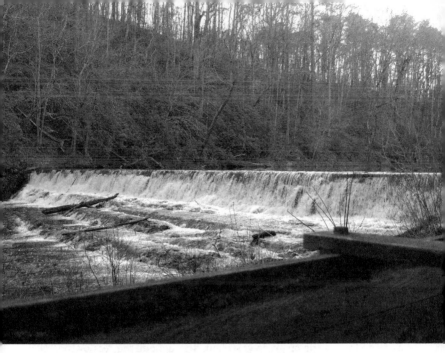

WATER RUSHES OVER THE MILLPOND DAM UPSTREAM OF TANNEHILL'S GRISTMILL.

The cemetery has been fenced off. Aside from one marked grave, a more modern burial, the gravesites are difficult to discern, marked only by rocks. About 60 slaves are believed to have been buried here. Slaves provided the primary labor for building and operating the furnaces.

Whichever way you return to the trail from the cemetery, you'll pick up the trail that follows the Old Bucksville Stage Road, a wagon route that connected the nearby Bucksville settlement to Montevallo. The furnace iron would continue on this route south to Montevallo, about 18 miles away, where it would be loaded on trains bound for the Confederate arsenal at Selma.

Heading north, the Stage Road crosses a succession of small hills before coming to an intersection with the Slave Quarters Trail. You will turn left here, along the route slaves walked from housing to the furnaces. However, you can also take a side trip by continuing straight to the rebuilt gristmill on Mill Creek.

The John Wesley Hall Grist Mill and Cotton Gin operated at this site from 1867 to 1931. This reconstruction was completed in 1976. It's worth a visit, if only to see the millpond and the wide waterfall it creates.

Retrace your steps to the Slave Quarters Trail and head southwest. Along the way, trees are identified with labels. The diversity of Alabama's forests is on display here. In this short stretch alone, there are so many species I lost count. There are at least five oak species: willow, post, water, red, and scarlet. There are American, winged, and slippery elms; loblolly and Virginia pines; cedar; hackberry; black cherry; black willow; black gum; sweet gum; and beech, to name a few. And it's worth remembering that all this land was once shorn of its timber to feed the furnaces.

Recross the creek and head back past the furnace and through the pioneer village to the parking area.

Nearby Attractions

While you're out this way, consider visiting a couple of landmark restaurants in Bessemer. **The Bright Star,** at 304 N. 19th St., serves Greek-style seafood and Southern vegetables (205-424-9444, **thebrightstar .com**). Having served patrons since 1907, it is Alabama's oldest family-owned restaurant and has received national accolades. The classic barbecue landmark **Bob Sykes Bar-B-Q,** at 1724 Ninth Ave. N., has been serving up smoked pork since 1957 (205-426-1400, **bobsykes.com**).

Directions

Tannehill Ironworks Historical State Park is located at 12632 Confederate Pkwy. in McCalla. Take I-20/I-59 to Exit 100 (Abernant/Bucksville) and follow the signs along Tannehill Parkway (about 2 miles), or take I-459 to Exit 1 (McCalla) and follow the signs along Eastern Valley Road (about 7 miles).

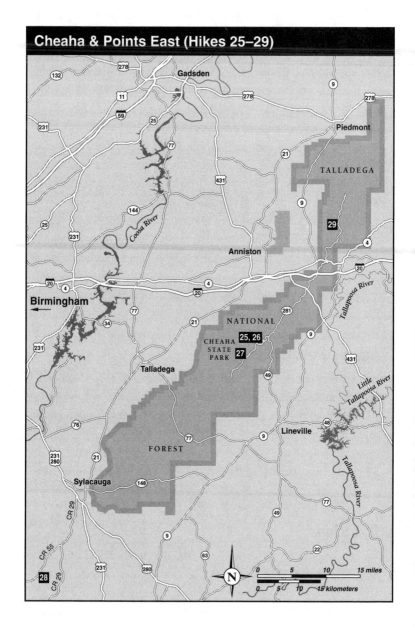

Cheaha & Points East (Hikes 25–29)

132

278

Gadsden

11

59

231

25

25

77

144

Coosa River

231

278

9

278

Piedmont

21

9

TALLADEGA

29

4

431

Anniston

20

4

4

20

Tallapoosa River

Birmingham

77

34

21

281

NATIONAL

25, 26

CHEAHA
STATE
PARK

27

9

431

231

Talladega

49

Little
Tallapoosa River

76

77

9

Lineville

48

FOREST

231
280

21

Sylacauga

148

9

49

Tallapoosa River

CR 29

28

CR 55

CR 29

231

280

9

63

77

22

0   5   10   15 miles

N

0   5   10   15 kilometers

Cheaha & Points East

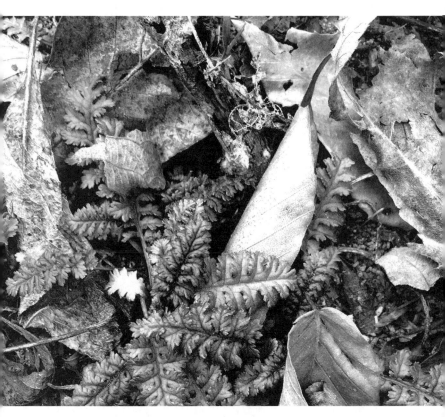

FERN FRONDS NESTLE AMONG THE LEAF LITTER ALONG THE PINHOTI TRAIL IN THE TALLADEGA NATIONAL FOREST. *(See Hike 29.)*

Cheaha & Points East Overview

THE HIKES IN THIS SECTION are concentrated in and around **Cheaha State Park,** which serves as a good introduction point and staging ground for further exploration, and which contains the highest point in Alabama, Mount Cheaha. At the Cheaha park store, you can pick up maps and get the latest trail information.

Aside from the Flagg Mountain hike, all of this section's hikes branch off the central artery of the Talladega National Forest, AL 281, or its unpaved northern extension, Forest Service Road 500, collectively known as the Talladega Scenic Drive or the Skyway Motorway.

If you want to make it a weekend of hiking, you can set up a base camp at the state park or in the national forest at the Pine Glen, Coleman Lake, or Turnipseed Campground (visit **www.fs.usda.gov /alabama** for more information).

East Alabama is also home to the **Pinhoti Trail,** the state's long-distance hiking trail and its connection to the Appalachian Trail (AT). This footpath starts on Flagg Mountain in the Weogufka State Forest and follows some roadways, then runs the length of the Talladega National Forest from Sylacauga to the Georgia line. More than 100 miles in Alabama are followed by about 200 miles of Pinhoti in Georgia on which you can eventually connect to the AT. Shelters and primitive camping are available at US Forest Service campsites at Pine Glen and Coleman Lake in Cleburne County. In July 2014, the Forest Service published a new consolidated map of the Pinhoti Trail that includes the trails around Cheaha. For hikes that include the Pinhoti, see pages 206 and 229; for more information, see **pinhotitrailalliance.org.**

Obviously, there are a lot of recreational options in the area around **Anniston** (see next page), and I haven't even mentioned the water options you can find on the **Coosa** and **Tallapoosa Rivers** and their tributaries.

Other Area Attractions

Mount Cheaha may be the state's highest point, but it's just one high point among many in east Alabama. Here's a sampling:

ANNISTON MUSEUM OF NATURAL HISTORY AND BERMAN MUSEUM OF WORLD HISTORY Two great small museums kids will like, located next to each other in Anniston's Lagarde Park (at the intersection of AL 21 and US 431). The Museum of Natural History features dinosaurs, an Egyptian mummy, and displays on ecology and geology. The Berman Museum has guns and weapons galore, plus Asian and European art and American Indian items. More information: **annistonmuseum.org** and **bermanmuseum.org.**

CHIEF LADIGA TRAIL Stretching 33 miles from Anniston to the Georgia line, the Chief Ladiga Trail continues in Georgia as the Silver Comet Trail for a total of almost 100 miles to the outskirts of Atlanta. Paved with a mostly gentle grade, the route passes through several towns. There are campsites along the way. In one of its prettiest stretches, north of Piedmont, the rail-trail passes through the Talladega National Forest and crosses the Pinhoti Trail. More information: **chiefladigatrail.com.**

COLDWATER MOUNTAIN BIKING TRAILS A nationally recognized and still-expanding network of trails built by the International Mountain Biking Association on a 4,000-acre tract of mountaintop Forever Wild property near Anniston and Oxford. Choose from short beginner trails or long-distance advanced options. For more information, visit the Northeast Alabama Bicycle Association at **neaba.net** or the Forever Wild Land Trust at **alabamaforeverwild.com.**

MOUNTAIN LONGLEAF NATIONAL REFUGE One of the country's newest wildlife refuges, carved out of the old Fort McClellan army base near Anniston, Mountain Longleaf features old-growth and second-growth longleaf-pine forests. Established in 2003, the refuge allows public access, but not much has been developed as far as trails and facilities. Bains Gap Road passes through the refuge. Visit **fws .gov/southeast/mountainlongleaf** for more information.

25 Cheaha–Cave Creek– Pinhoti Trail Loop

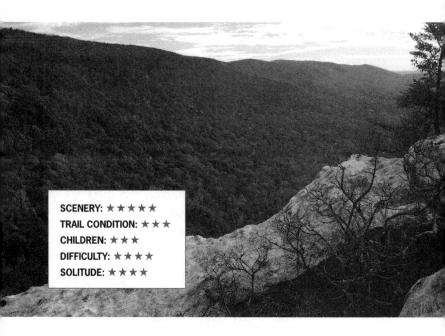

SCENERY: ★ ★ ★ ★ ★
TRAIL CONDITION: ★ ★ ★
CHILDREN: ★ ★ ★
DIFFICULTY: ★ ★ ★ ★
SOLITUDE: ★ ★ ★ ★

GPS TRAILHEAD COORDINATES: N33° 28.286' W85° 48.385'

DISTANCE & CONFIGURATION: 6.7-mile loop

HIKING TIME: 5.5 hours

HIGHLIGHTS: Tunnels of rhododendron, views of surrounding mountain ridges, the rocky overlook at McDill Point, the wreckage of a single-engine plane crash, and monuments dedicating the Cheaha Wilderness and the Pinhoti Trail, Alabama's principal long-distance wilderness hiking trail and its connection to the Appalachian Trail.

ELEVATION: Hike begins at 1,933' and reaches a high point of 2,340'.

ACCESS: Every day, all year. Camping permitted.

MAPS: USFS *Pinhoti Trail Map;* less-detailed hiking maps also available at Cheaha State Park

FACILITIES: Information kiosk at the trailhead, which is a short distance from Cheaha State Park, where all your basic amenities are available

WHEELCHAIR ACCESS: None

COMMENTS: This hike is rocky and rugged in places. Wear boots. Bring plenty of water.

CONTACT: www.fs.usda.gov/alabama; check "Know Before You Go."

Overview

This hike, which starts in Cheaha State Park and ventures into the Talladega National Forest's Cheaha Wilderness, offers a contrast between the two flanks of the same mountain—an eastern side with gentle contours and rich vegetation and a western flank that is rockier, with dramatic dropoffs and overlooks, including the landmark McDill Point. The hike also includes a stretch of the Pinhoti Trail, Alabama's connector to the Appalachian Trail.

Route Details

This is a rigorous daylong hike. If you're making it in the fall, get started early. There is no shortcut. You'll start on the Cave Creek Trail, going about 3 miles to the south, then come back to the north 4 miles on the Pinhoti Trail to the trailhead, a total distance that includes a side trip to the McDill Point overlook.

When we hiked it, we started the trail with a nice group from Vestavia Hills whose party included some younger children. They decided to hike the loop in the opposite direction. We met up with them on the Pinhoti side near McDill Point. There was some dissension in that group about whether to turn back or make the whole loop. I wasn't much help because I wasn't sure how far we'd come and how far we had to go. They continued on. When we finished, they were nowhere in sight and it was getting dark. I trust they made it out, but I fear some of the young ones on the trip may have permanently sworn off hiking.

All this is to say, this hike is not for young children or the novice hiker. I sympathized with the leader of the other expedition, because I've often been in the position of pushing people beyond their comfort level and operating on inadequate information. Seeing it from the outside, it occurred to me that I ought to include a warning in this book: Try to plan a suitable hike for your party. Once you're too far out, it's not like you can call a cab.

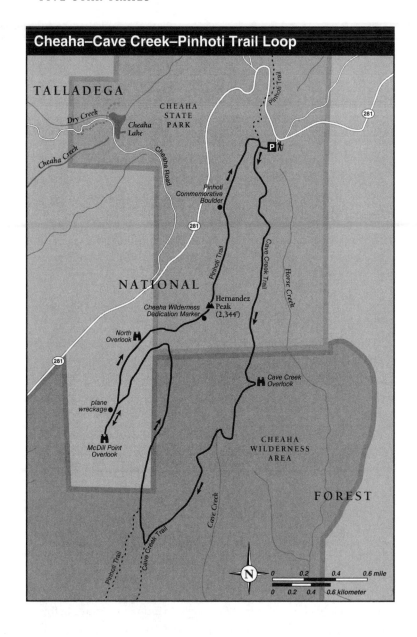

Cheaha–Cave Creek–Pinhoti Trail Loop

TALLADEGA

Dry Creek

Cheaha Creek

Cheaha Lake

CHEAHA STATE PARK

Cheaha Road

Pinhoti Trail

281

281

Pinhoti Commemorative Boulder

Pinhoti Trail

Cave Creek Trail

Horse Creek

NATIONAL

Cheaha Wilderness Dedication Marker

Hernandez Peak (2,344')

North Overlook

281

Cave Creek Overlook

plane wreckage

McDill Point Overlook

CHEAHA WILDERNESS AREA

FOREST

Pinhoti Trail

Cave Creek Trail

Cave Creek

N

| 0 | 0.2 | 0.4 | 0.6 mile |

| 0 | 0.2 | 0.4 | 0.6 kilometer |

Shortly after leaving the parking area, a sign points to the right for a connector trail to the Pinhoti—this is the connector you'll return by. For now, head left on the Cave Creek Trail. This is a lovely trail to hike in the fall because of the contrast between the evergreen rhododendrons and the changing red and yellow leaves of the plentiful maple trees. The rhododendrons bloom in late spring and early summer, other good times to take this loop.

This eastern flank on the mountain feels sheltered and secluded. The Cave Creek Trail is unblazed, but it is well worn, and for the purposes of this loop hike, red arrows mark the way at confusing junctions.

Along the way, you cross several wet-weather drainages. They were, for the most part, dry when we hiked in the fall but should be pretty to see in the winter and spring.

Eventually you come to an outcropping that offers a nice view. Then the trail switches back to climb the mountain. You pass through a pine forest and come upon a fire ring and campsite. Follow the red arrow to the right. Shortly you'll pass a pretty little spring-fed, rhododendron-sheltered stream. This is Cave Creek.

Crossing it, we happened to notice crawfish scuttling about along the rocks in the clear water. It's a wonder that so high on the mountain in this tiny water source you'd have a thriving population of aquatic critters.

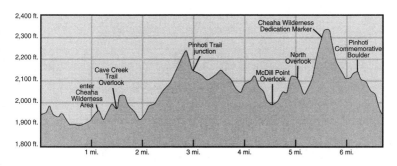

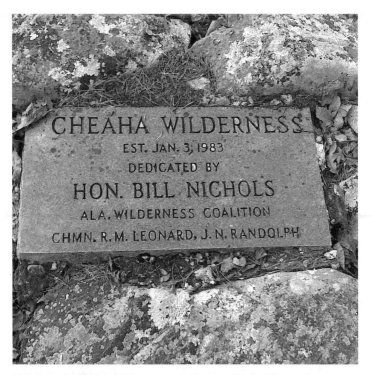

THIS PLAQUE MARKS THE DEDICATION OF THE CHEAHA WILDERNESS.

After the creek comes a pretty nice climb to the connector trail to the Pinhoti. About now it begins to feel like you've come a long way.

The connector takes you over the ridge, through a collection of boulders, and down to where you pick up the Pinhoti, which is blazed blue. The Pinhoti is also marked with diamond-shaped metallic signs with a turkey track in the middle.

This next stretch is rocky and rough, but it has great views. Soon you'll see signs offering you a side trip to the McDill Point overlook. Take the trip. It's well worth it. The point is a rocky outcropping that overlooks a gulf of woodlands. Looking off to the south and west, all you see is the unbroken forest of the Talladega Mountains. Cheaha has nice overlooks that are easier to get to, but this is one of the best scenic spots in the state of Alabama because you have to earn it.

The trip back to the trailhead on the Pinhoti is a little more than 2 miles. Along the way, notice rock formations that include layers of crystallized rock. That rock was squeezed under tremendous pressure during the continental collisions that formed the Appalachian Mountains; it "cooked" into quartz.

There are a couple of other landmarks along the path. One is a granite marker commemorating the dedication of the Cheaha Wilderness on January 3, 1983. The other is a huge stone boulder with a bronze plaque marking the connection of the Pinhoti Trail to the Appalachian Trail. Advocates hope that one day the Pinhoti will be officially dedicated as part of the Appalachian Trail, which now begins in north Georgia at Springer Mountain. After all, if you're going to hike the length of the Appalachian Mountains, you ought to start at the southernmost mountain, which is Alabama's Flagg Mountain (see page 222).

During your return trip, the trail crosses and recrosses a jeep road. Make sure to keep following the blue blazes and retrace the path to the parking area at the Cheaha Trailhead. And remember that close to the end of the hike, you'll leave the Pinhoti and follow a short connector trail, marked by signs pointing to parking and the Cave Creek Trail, as the Pinhoti continues on to the Blue Mountain Shelter.

Directions

Take I-20 East to Exit 191 (US 431). Take a right onto US 431 South. After 3.5 miles, take a right onto CR 131, following the signs to Cheaha State Park. After half a mile, take a left onto AL 281 (also known as the Talladega Scenic Drive), heading south. Continue 12 miles until you reach the Cheaha and Cave Creek Trailhead. If you reach the Cheaha State Park entrance, you've gone half a mile too far south.

26

Cheaha State Park:
Bald Rock & Pulpit Rock

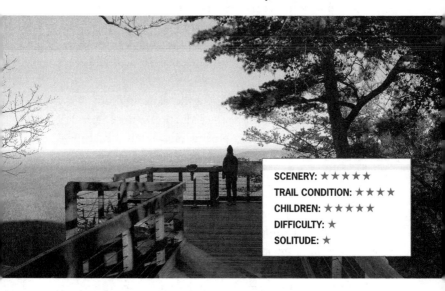

SCENERY: ★ ★ ★ ★ ★
TRAIL CONDITION: ★ ★ ★ ★
CHILDREN: ★ ★ ★ ★ ★
DIFFICULTY: ★
SOLITUDE: ★

GPS TRAILHEAD COORDINATES: N33° 29.484' W85° 48.675' (Bald Rock Trailhead), N33° 29.046' W85° 48.896' (Pulpit Rock Trailhead), N33° 29.128' W85° 48.525' (Bunker Tower)

DISTANCE & CONFIGURATION: 0.5-mile out-and-back to Bald Rock; 1-mile out-and-back to Pulpit Rock

HIKING TIME: 20 minutes

HIGHLIGHTS: Tremendous views from the highest point(s) in Alabama

ELEVATION: 2,160' at Pulpit Rock Overlook, 2,330' at Bald Rock Overlook, 2,407' at Bunker Tower

ACCESS: Open daily, 7 a.m.–sunset; park store open 8 a.m.–9 p.m. Day-use fees: $2 for children and adults over age 6, $1 for adults over age 62.

MAPS: Available at Cheaha State Park store and the website below.

FACILITIES: Camp store, restaurant, swimming and fishing lake, mountain biking trails, Indian-artifact museum, cabins, motel, developed and primitive campsites

WHEELCHAIR ACCESS: The Doug Ghee Interpretive Trail to Bald Rock is wheelchair-accessible.

COMMENTS: At the endpoints of both suggested hikes, there are steep and rocky dropoffs. Keep an eye on children. While it's thrilling to venture out on the rocks for a view, it's important to stay safe.

CONTACT: 256-488-5111 or 800-610-5801, **alapark.com/cheaharesort**

Overview

Everyone needs to make a pilgrimage to the highest point in Alabama: Mount Cheaha's peak, in Cheaha State Park. Climb the stone observation tower, built by the Civilian Conservation Corps, for a 360-degree view. Take advantage of short hikes to Pulpit Rock or Bald Rock to get to mountain's edge. It can be crowded, but it's worth it to see the fall leaves. Head to the mountains and cool off in the summer. A nice intro to the outdoors, the state park can also be a staging ground for more hiking and waterfall pilgrimages in the surrounding Talladega National Forest and Cheaha Wilderness.

Route Details

When I posted pictures of an autumn trip to Cheaha State Park, several people asked, "Where were you?!"—a question with the subtext "Surely you traveled far from Alabama to see something this magnificent."

Not that I blame them. We had the same reaction. As we climbed and twisted along the scenic parkway that winds its way through the Talladega Mountain ridges, we felt as if we'd pulled onto the Blue Ridge Parkway, but we were just a little more than an hour away from Birmingham, uphill from Anniston. In the fall, the green forested mountainsides are awash with reds, yellows, and browns. Scenic overlooks offer grand views, largely undisturbed ridges and valleys, and the wide Coosa Valley.

Cheaha State Park itself comprises 2,799 acres, but it's within the 235,000-acre Talladega District of the Talladega National Forest. Its highest point, Mount Cheaha, rises 2,407 feet above sea level, and throughout the park and in the surrounding forest, rocky outcroppings offer dramatic views.

You don't have to hike to experience those views. You can enjoy them from the state-park restaurant, sipping a beverage if you like. At the other extreme, miles and miles of nearby trails will take you deep into the wilderness. But for the purposes of this entry, I'm

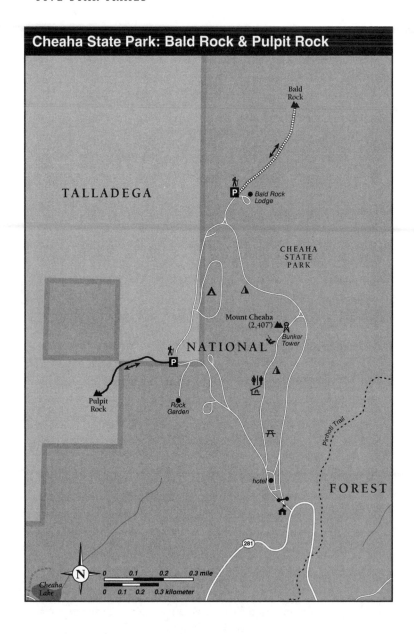

Cheaha State Park: Bald Rock & Pulpit Rock

Bald Rock

TALLADEGA

P Bald Rock
Lodge

CHEAHA
STATE
PARK

Mount Cheaha
(2,407)

Bunker
Tower

NATIONAL

P

Pulpit
Rock

Rock
Garden

Pinhoti Trail

hotel

FOREST

281

N

| 0 | 0.1 | 0.2 | 0.3 mile |

| 0 | 0.1 | 0.2 | 0.3 kilometer |

Cheaha
Lake

suggesting three easy stops at Cheaha State Park that give you a taste of northeast Alabama.

After you enter the park, a good first stop is the Bunker Tower, built in the 1930s by the Civilian Conservation Corps as part of the original improvements to the park. Climb the stairs to the top of the tower; from the observation deck, you can survey the state, in all directions, from its highest point. The base of the tower includes a CCC museum, recently reopened.

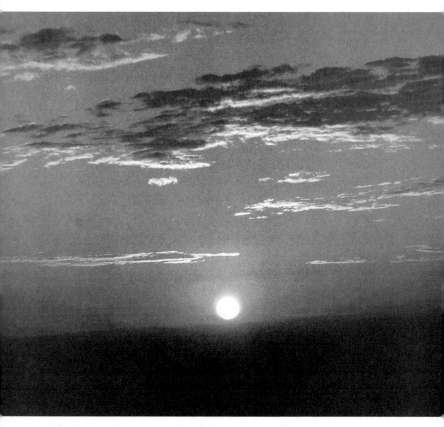

A SUNSET VIEW FROM ATOP ALABAMA'S HIGHEST MOUNTAIN

There are picnic and play areas nearby if needed. Because the road system is a one-way loop, you continue around and circle back to the main park road on your way to the Bald Rock Boardwalk, also known as the Doug Ghee Interpretive Trail.

This boardwalk trail begins at the Bald Rock Lodge, also built by the CCC. It served as the original hotel at the park and is still used as a group rental lodge and conference center. The boardwalk includes interpretive signage that helps give you the lay of the land. At the end, you'll have northwest views of the Coosa Valley, Oxford, and Anniston.

For a more woodsy walk to an even better view, make your way to the Pulpit Rock Trail. It features dogwoods blooming around Easter, mountain laurels in May, and of course fall color. This walk is 1 easy mile in total, though coming back requires a little bit of a climb. And you'll want to watch your step on the rocks. The trail is marked with red blazes and is easy to follow until the area approaching the rock outcropping. But worry not; there's really only one way to the end of the promontory. Once you're there, you have great views to the south and the forested Talladega Mountains—some of the best views in Alabama.

Hold on to kids around here. These are real cliffs with 70- to 100-foot drops.

On the way out, it's worth stopping at the park restaurant for the view and, if it's cold, maybe some hot chocolate.

Directions

Take I-20 East to Exit 191 (US 431). Turn right onto US 431 South. After 3.5 miles, turn right onto CR 131, following the signs to Cheaha State Park. After 0.5 mile, take a left onto AL 281 (Talladega Scenic Drive), heading south. Continue 12 miles until you reach the park entrance.

27

Chinnabee Silent Trail

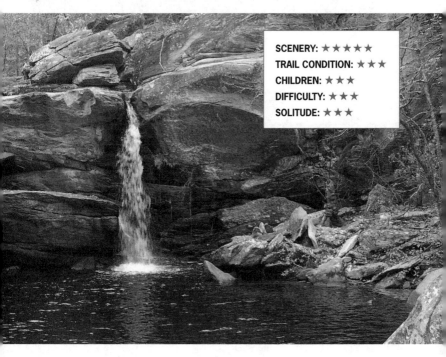

SCENERY: ★ ★ ★ ★ ★
TRAIL CONDITION: ★ ★ ★
CHILDREN: ★ ★ ★
DIFFICULTY: ★ ★ ★
SOLITUDE: ★ ★ ★

GPS TRAILHEAD COORDINATES: N33° 26.650' W85° 50.473'

DISTANCE & CONFIGURATION: 6.4-mile out-and-back

HIKING TIME: 4 hours

HIGHLIGHTS: Waterfalls at Cheaha Falls and Devil's Den; longleaf ridges and hardwood hollows

ELEVATION: 1,150' at start, 850' at low point

ACCESS: Every day, all year. Camping permitted.

MAPS: USFS *Pinhoti Trail Map;* less-detailed hiking maps also available at Cheaha State Park

FACILITIES: The Cheaha Falls Shelter for campers is on the trail, on a high point uphill from the falls.

WHEELCHAIR ACCESS: None

COMMENTS: Segments of this trail and the surrounding landscape along Cheaha Creek near Devil's Den sustained heavy damage from flooding during the summer of 2013.

CONTACT: US Forest Service, Talladega District, 256-362-2909, **pa_alabama@fs.fed.us**, **www.fs.usda.gov/detail/alabama/about-forest/districts**

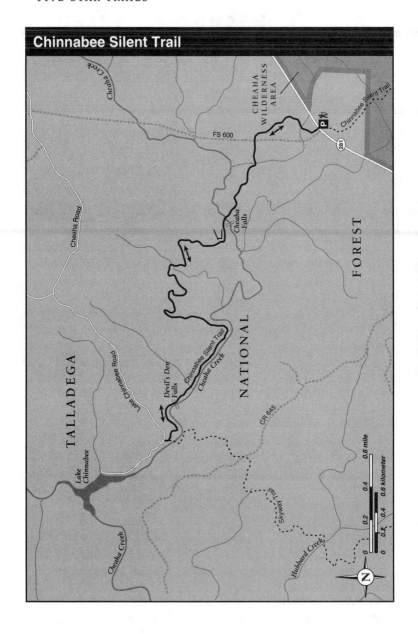

Chinnabee Silent Trail

Overview

This out-and-back trek, a total of 6 miles on the Chinnabee Silent Trail, hits at least two of Cheaha's scenic highlights: Cheaha Falls and a magnificent series of cascading falls known as Devil's Den. In addition, you'll get views of surrounding ridges from high pine slopes and fall color in hardwood draws.

Route Details

You'll start at the Scenic Drive and hike about a mile to Cheaha Creek, visit Cheaha Falls, and then hike for about a mile and a half up and down draws until you rejoin the creek. After a half-mile, the creek makes a series of beautiful drops known as Devil's Den. The trail after Cheaha Falls is less traveled and a little harder to follow, and the last half-mile to Devil's Den shows damage from the floods of 2013. But for those who press on, the sights at Devil's Den are well worth the trek.

One of Alabama's classic trails, the Chinnabee Silent Trail is 6 miles in total, running from the Lake Chinnabee Recreation Area (750 feet in elevation) to Caney Head atop Talladega Mountain (2,100 feet). *Silent* is a tribute to Boy Scout Troop 29 from the Alabama Institute for Deaf and Blind in Talladega, who constructed the trail in 1977.

The particular segment I'm recommending doesn't reach Lake Chinnabee Recreation Area, which was closed due to damage caused

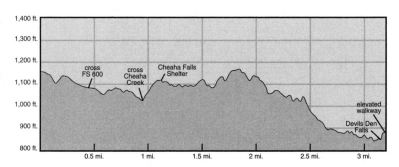

by flooding in the summer of 2013 but has since reopened for day use. It also leaves off the steep climb to the top of Talladega Mountain.

To get to the trailhead, take the Scenic Drive south past the entrance to Cheaha State Park for 3 miles, to a parking lot on the left side of the road. To begin the hike, you cross the Scenic Drive on foot, following the hiking trail signs toward Cheaha Falls.

You may see some references to the Chinnabee Silent Trail being marked with blue blazes. When we hiked the trail, those blue blazes had long since faded to white.

The hike traverses a draw, then crosses Forest Service Road 600 before proceeding deeper into the woods. There is nice fall color on this stretch. As you approach Cheaha Falls, spur trails shoot off in several directions toward campsites near the falls. The real trail cuts across Cheaha Creek upstream of the falls and heads up the ridge toward the Cheaha Falls Shelter.

Apparently, there used to be a bridge here. When we crossed the creek, it was easy to traverse a rock ledge, but in wetter weather this might require a little fording.

But before all that, you'll want to follow your ears downstream to Cheaha Falls. The creek here has carved out a crude amphitheater in the rock, and at the base of the falls is a swimming hole, which looked like it would be a cool rush in the summer.

Instead, we clambered around the rocks for the right view, then took in the sights and sounds. For a simple 2-mile hike with young children, you could turn around right here and head back to the car. But there are more impressive sights to see if you press on.

Cross the creek and head up the ridge to the Cheaha Falls Shelter. This would be a great place to camp, perched up on a piney ridge with great views of the ridges to the east and in close proximity to the falls.

When we arrived in the early afternoon, it was unoccupied, but on our return a couple of parties had set up camp. A couple of other groups were camping down by the falls.

From the shelter atop the ridge, the trail heads off into the woods away from Cheaha Creek. You cross pine ridges and dip down into hardwood draws with great fall color for about a mile and a half before finally rejoining Cheaha Creek. This stretch seems longer. Impatient to see the creek again, I was nervous that we'd picked up another trail and were headed in the wrong direction. Eventually, though, you'll follow the flow of a drainage back to the creek.

When you finally rejoin it, you encounter a stretch of trail that is beaten up and damaged from debris from the 2013 flooding. Along the creek, webs of dead sticks and leaves and small trees are wrapped around the trees and entangled in the brush. It looks like the creek rose 8 feet above its normal level.

Just keep in mind that you don't cross the creek, and you'll be fine following the trail. Proceed downstream and soon you'll hear the rush of water as the creek drops into a canyon. This dramatic series of stairstep falls is known as Devil's Den. The creek drops significantly in elevation in a short stretch, forming a dozen shelves and drops along the way.

It's a lovely sight and a lovely sound thanks to the enclosing walls of the canyon.

Find the right vantage point and take it in. It's one of those places where you think about the force of water over time. You can continue down the trail a bit and get a view of the falls from an elevated wooden walkway. We turned around here.

The hike back goes all too quickly.

Directions

Take I-20 East to Exit 191 (US 431). Turn right onto US 431 South. After 3.5 miles, turn right onto CR 131, following the signs to Cheaha State Park. After 0.5 mile, take a left onto AL 281 (Talladega Scenic Drive), heading south. After 12 miles, you'll reach the entrance to Cheaha State Park. Continue past the park entrance for 3 miles on 281. You'll find a parking lot on the left side of road. Cross to the opposite side of the road to begin the hike.

28

Flagg Mountain:
The Southernmost Appalachian

SCENERY: ★ ★ ★ ★ ★
TRAIL CONDITION: ★ ★ ★ ★ ★
CHILDREN: ★ ★ ★
DIFFICULTY: ★ ★
SOLITUDE: ★

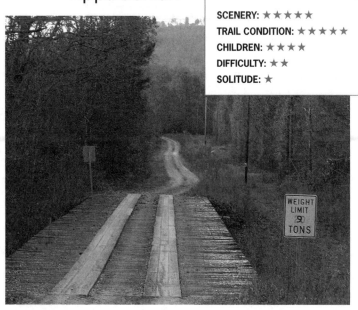

GPS TRAILHEAD COORDINATES: N32° 59.107' W86° 21.243'

DISTANCE & CONFIGURATION: 3.7-mile loop

HIKING TIME: 3 hours

HIGHLIGHTS: Historic stone fire tower built by the Civilian Conservation Corps, mature longleaf pines, unique fauna, and great views from the southernmost Appalachian Mountain

ELEVATION: 750' at trailhead; 1,142' at fire tower

ACCESS: Daily; stay out of all buildings on the property.

MAPS: USGS *Flagg Mountain*

FACILITIES: 2 fire rings and campsites along the trail, 1 picnic table

WHEELCHAIR ACCESS: None

COMMENTS: Fall is a great time to visit Flagg Mountain, but bear in mind that the property is surrounded by a wildlife-management area and by property leased to hunting clubs. It's a good idea to wear orange and take care to stay on the trail. You can peek in the windows of the fire tower, but it's closed to the public, so please don't enter.

CONTACT: Not applicable

Overview

If you really want to hike the Appalachian Mountains, you need to start at Flagg Mountain, which, at 1,152 feet above sea level, is the chain's southernmost peak. This introductory hike offers great views and modest climbs up and down the draws on the mountain's flanks. On the summit itself, you can see the remains of what was to be a state park, including a stone fire tower built by the Civilian Conservation Corps during the Depression. You also see the surrounding country: the foothills falling off to the coastal plain and the mountains, including Cheaha, the state's highest peak, rising in the northeast.

Route Details

This hike through the Weogufka State Forest on Flagg Mountain starts from the northern trailhead on CCC Camp Road and makes a semicircle around the mountaintop before rejoining CCC Camp Road at the southern trailhead. You then follow the dirt road back up and over the mountain to the northern trailhead. The hike has some climb and descent but nothing overly challenging. At less than 4 miles long, it requires moderate effort. The trail is well marked with yellow blazes, thanks to the Alabama Hiking Trail Society.

This destination is not well known right now, but word is getting out. It's a draw for several reasons, one being its history. Flagg Mountain was a work site for the New Deal's Civilian Conservation Corps, a government program that put unemployed men back to work building public-works projects. The work of the CCC can be seen at various state parks, including Cheaha and Oak Mountain. Flagg Mountain was to have been a state park, too, but Alabama never came up with the money to develop it. The cabins and other structures built by the CCC were abandoned for decades until a group of Coosa County volunteers stepped in and started restoring them. It's an ongoing process, and visitors are asked to refrain from entering the structures.

Another reason Flagg Mountain is of note is that it serves as the southern trailhead of the Pinhoti Trail, a long-distance hiking trail that

Flagg Mountain: The Southernmost Appalachian

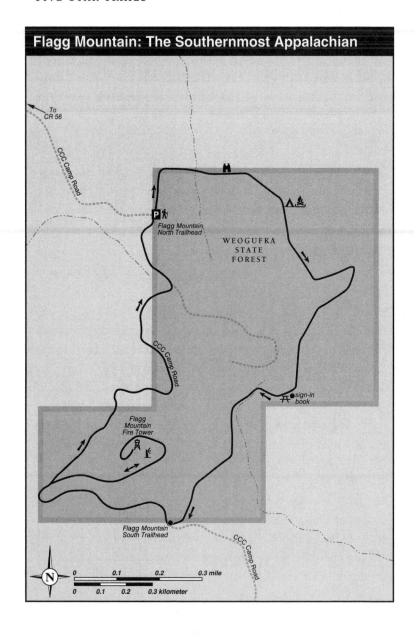

To
CR 56

CCC Camp Road

P Flagg Mountain
North Trailhead

WEOGUFKA
STATE
FOREST

CCC Camp Road

sign-in
book

Flagg
Mountain
Fire Tower

Flagg Mountain
South Trailhead

CCC Camp Road

N

| 0 | | 0.1 | | 0.2 | | 0.3 mile |

0   0.1   0.2   0.3 kilometer

traverses the Talladega National Forest and continues into Georgia. At 335 miles long, the Pinhoti serves as a connector to the Appalachian Trail. It would take some serious persuasion, but advocates dream of the day when Flagg Mountain is officially designated the southern terminus of the AT. Currently, the AT runs 2,181 miles, from Springer Mountain in north Georgia to Mount Katahdin in Maine.

But we're getting ahead of ourselves. Today we're going to appreciate the virtues of Flagg Mountain itself.

The trailhead is well marked with a green-and-yellow diamond-shaped sign with the Alabama Hiking Trails logo on it. Coming from Lay Dam Road, it will be on the left side of CCC Camp Road about half-way up the mountain, a little less than a mile after you cross a weight-limited, one-lane wooden bridge. A couple of trails collide here. For this hike, you want to follow the yellow blazes.

Proceeding into the woods, you'll notice a pattern that will repeat itself on this hike. At the higher elevations, you're in a mixed pine–hardwood forest with a healthy presence of longleaf pine. Then the trail descends a draw in the mountainside and the pines disappear. At the base of the draw you'll find a little creek, often sheltered by beech trees. Like other hardwoods, the beeches turn colors in the fall but hold on to their copper-colored leaves. They're easy to identify in winter.

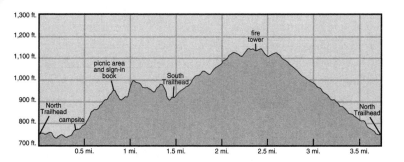

As you climb out of the draw to the next ridge, the pines return. This trail is also sprinkled with evergreen American holly and rhododendron.

A little more than a half-mile into this hike, you make one of these ascents, and through the trees you get a glimpse of the next mountain ridge in the near distance. When I reached this point, I thought about what it would feel like if I were setting off to hike the Appalachians. With fresh legs and the gentle humps of low mountains before me, I had an urge to do it.

Shortly after this hint of a view, you'll see a metal fire ring and a trailside campsite. On my hike, as I was surveying the campsite, a commotion commenced high in the trees above me. I looked up to see a large turkey making an awkward B-52–like glide from his roost, away from me and down deeper into the forest.

Pressing on, you soon reach a junction with a white-blazed trail that heads back to the north trailhead. Continue to follow the yellow blazes, enjoying views of the valley below. You'll cross an old logging road and ascend; at 1 mile into the hike, you'll see a trail sign, a picnic table, a fire pit, and, at least in winter, a glorious view.

Leaving the picnic area, the trail goes downhill ever so briefly, then cuts sharply left. Just make sure you're still following the yellow-blazed trail. Continuing, I came to what I'll call my cathedral moment. This was an early Sunday morning, and I had just checked my watch and calculated that I wasn't going to make it back to Birmingham for church. Looking up, I noticed two huge longleaf pines on either side of the trail. It's rare that you see them that large nowadays. As I passed them, I had the distinct sense that I was entering a sanctuary. The trail dropped down to a spring-fed creek sheltered by a grove of large beech trees. In this sheltered cove, it was extraordinarily quiet. Against the hillside of fallen leaves lay moss-covered boulders. The columns of bare trees reached to the blue ceiling of sky. Across the little creek there was an unexpected evergreen canebrake and, as the creek fell away down the mountain, a robust growth of rhododendron, also unusual this far south in Alabama. Taking it in,

I let out an involuntary whoop of joy. I knew that I was where I was supposed to be at that moment on that day.

With a spring in my step, I continued on. Less than half a mile later, at the 1.5-mile mark on the hike, I reached the southern trailhead at CCC Camp Road.

To finish the hike from here, turn right and proceed uphill back toward the north. At the top of the ridge, the road forks. The right fork continues uphill to the mountaintop fire tower. The left fork continues downhill back to the northern trailhead. For the full experience, follow that right fork. The great views you've had along the way continue to get better as you approach the peak. On a clear day, you can see Alabama Power's Gaston steam plant to the north, Cheaha to the east-northeast, and farms and woodlands in the valley below.

At the summit is the CCC-constructed fire tower, a twin to the Bunker Tower on Cheaha. Adjoining the tower is a small stone lodge building with a big fireplace, above which hangs a large American flag. The lease to this building is held by the heroic group of locals who have put a great deal of effort into preserving the CCC structures on the mountain. The structures are closed to the public. The stairs in the fire tower are original and may be hazardous to climb.

Still, this is a great spot to think about the underused assets we have in this state, the work that has gone into building and restoring them, and the potential we have if we'd work together to make the best use of them.

With that in mind, follow the road back down to the fork and return downhill to the northern trailhead.

Nearby Attractions

In Weogufka, the community at the crossroads of County Roads 29 and 56, there is a collection of historic buildings, including **Caperton's Old South General Store & Pawn Shoppe** (256-249-9100), built in 1853. The store sells knives, ammo, snacks and drinks, and Confederate memorabilia.

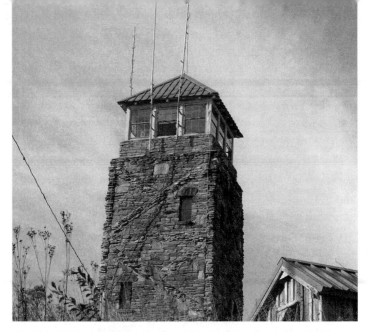

THE CCC FIRE TOWER IS NICE TO LOOK AT, BUT DON'T TRY TO GET INSIDE.

Just off US 280 in Sylacauga is the **Imerys–Gantt's Quarry Observation Site,** open daily, 9 a.m.–4 p.m. The site is 0.3 mile off US 280 on Fayetteville Highway (watch for the directional signs on 280). White marble mined in Sylacauga was used in the Lincoln Memorial, the Washington Monument, and the US Supreme Court building.

Directions

From Birmingham, you can take either US 280 East or I-65 South. If you're searching for directions online, use the term "Weogufka State Forest." Heading east on US 280 in Sylacauga, turn right onto County 29 (Coaling Road). After 8 miles, at the intersection in the Weogufka community, turn right onto CR 55 (Lay Dam Road). Continue 5.8 miles. Past the intersection with CR 56, look for a left turn onto CCC Camp Road, a dirt road that takes you into the woods. About a mile in, you'll cross a one-lane wooden bridge. The trailhead is less than a mile after that on the left side of the road, marked with a yellow-and-green diamond-shaped sign. Park on the right shoulder, just uphill from the trailhead.

29 Pinhoti Trail:
Lower Shoal Shelter Section

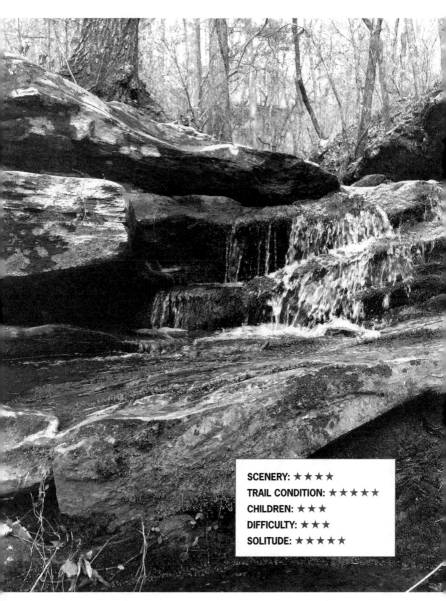

SCENERY: ★ ★ ★ ★
TRAIL CONDITION: ★ ★ ★ ★ ★
CHILDREN: ★ ★ ★
DIFFICULTY: ★ ★ ★
SOLITUDE: ★ ★ ★ ★ ★

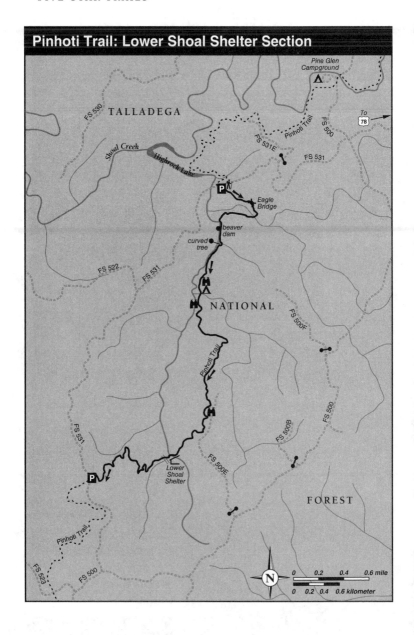

Pinhoti Trail: Lower Shoal Shelter Section

GPS TRAILHEAD COORDINATES: N33° 42.825' W85° 37.007' (Highrock Lake–FS 531 Trailhead), N33° 41.434', W85° 37.127' (FS 531 South Trailhead)

DISTANCE & CONFIGURATION: 4.4-mile point-to-point; requires a shuttle

HIKING TIME: 5 hours

HIGHLIGHTS: Meandering creeks, spring wildflowers, floodplain forest, high pine forests with nice views, Lower Shoal Shelter and waterfall

ACCESS: Always open

ELEVATION: 900' at Highrock Lake–FS 531 Trailhead; 1,280' at the FS 531 South Trailhead

MAPS: Available at the Pinhoti Trail Alliance website (see below)

FACILITIES: Lower Shoal Shelter

WHEELCHAIR ACCESS: None

COMMENTS: Consider calling the Forest Service before you go to find out about conditions, including any prescribed burns in the area. Don't try this section after heavy rain or if heavy rain is predicted, because creek crossings would be hazardous and FS 531 around the Highrock Lake Trailhead can experience dangerous flooding conditions.

CONTACT: US Forest Service, Shoal Creek Ranger District, 256-463-2272, **www.fs.usda .gov/alabama;** Pinhoti Trail Alliance, **pinhotitrailalliance.org**

Overview

This stretch of the Pinhoti serves as a nice introduction to less-traveled sections of the trail in the Shoal Creek Ranger District of the Talladega National Forest north of I-20. In 5 miles, you walk along clear, meandering streams and floodplain forest, then climb to high pine-forest ridges. There are plenty of wildflowers and even a

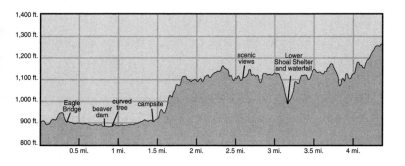

little waterfall at the Lower Shoal Shelter, a spot for backpackers to stop and camp. To make the hike, you'll need a car shuttle.

Route Details

I hiked this route in late March as part of a longer Boy Scout overnight expedition from the Pine Glen Campground to the Pinhoti Trailhead at Forest Service (FS) Road 500, just off US 78. It was difficult to choose a particular section to recommend, because I'm fond of multiple sections of the Pinhoti in this Cleburne County stretch of the Talladega National Forest.

I like the landscape, the relative solitude, and the convenience. If you look at an Alabama road map, it will show AL 281 (the Talladega Scenic Drive that goes up to Cheaha) ending at US 78, but that road actually continues, unpaved, into the national forest, becoming FS 500. The gravel road was cut by Civilian Conservation Corps crews in the 1930s. There are two developed campgrounds along this road: Coleman Lake to the north and Pine Glen about halfway to Coleman Lake. The Pinhoti runs north–south, roughly parallel to FS 500, and can be accessed at either campground or by a trailhead at the beginning of FS 500. In addition, the Pinhoti crosses smaller Forest Service roads at several points.

The stretch I'm suggesting begins in the north, where the Pinhoti crosses FS 531 near Highrock Lake and proceeds south to the Pinhoti–FS 531 South crossing. As you come north on FS 500, FS 531 branches off to the left. After 0.8 mile, watch carefully for red Pinhoti mileage signs on either side of the road. Park one car on the shoulder here, making sure not to block the road. Continue on FS 531 for 2.8 miles, until you reach the next Pinhoti crossing, near Highrock Lake. This is also known as the Drain Pipe Bridge crossing, because the road crosses a creek and a bridge. Don't try this hike if there has been heavy rain or if heavy rain is predicted—some creeks on the trail would be difficult to cross, plus this stretch of road can flood. Park off the road and away from low spots.

Take the Pinhoti south. A sign on the trail gives the mileage to the Lower Shoal Shelter as 4 miles and to FS 531 South as 5 miles (that's where you parked your shuttle car). You'll be following blue blazes on the trees, sometimes accompanied by diamond-shaped metallic Pinhoti signs.

The hike begins in low, wet forest, where beech trees cling to their copper leaves in winter and plenty of wildflowers emerge in the spring. Shortly you cross a sturdy wooden bridge built as part of an Eagle Scout project with the support of the Appalachian Trail Club of Alabama and Walmart. It's a good place to think about how much you owe to the volunteers who maintain these trails.

The trail tends to be well worn, but as it crosses a flat floodplain bottom, there aren't a lot of blazes. Two-tenths of a mile past the Eagle Bridge, you come to a large stream about 20 feet across. This can be a modestly tricky crossing if the water is flowing at normal levels. It can be hazardous when the water is high. We made our way across stepping from rock to rock, though at least one person in our party got a boot full of water and another lost balance and dropped a cell phone in the stream.

About a mile into the hike, which takes you along the creek, we spied a large beaver dam that created a large, wide backup of water. Beyond that, as the trail climbs a rise, an oddly bent tree to the right of the trail offers a nice place to sit. And about a mile and a half into the hike, a smaller creek crossing, about 10 feet wide, poses a challenge.

Once you're across, take note of a campsite with flat ground and plenty of water nearby. After the campsite and a creek crossing, the trail gains elevation, offering views of the floodplain forest below. The trees appear to be growing exceedingly tall as they race for the sun. When we were here in the early spring, there was almost no understory either. The Talladega National Forest is managed with an active regimen of prescribed burns, controlled forest fires that burn away fallen timber, simulating the natural cycle and creating a forest

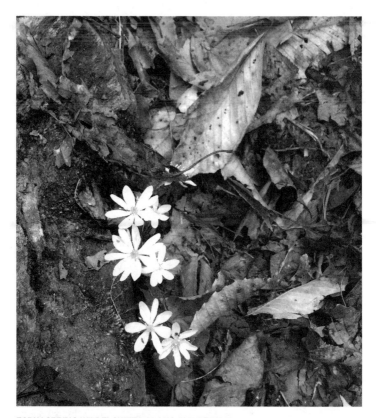

EARLY-SPRING WILDFLOWERS ALONG THE PINHOTI

that looks more like it would naturally when lightning-sparked wild-fires burned unchecked across the landscape.

The effects of these fires are more evident as you follow the trail up to higher elevations, where tall pines preside over a grassy understory. It's quiet here, away from the leaf crunch and up where the wind is a little stiffer. One of the joys of this part of the forest is that rippling ridges separate you from any sign of civilization. Aside from the occasional airplane, there is no detectable human noise. You hike along over 1,100 feet in elevation for a good stretch, enjoying the grasses, birdsong, and emerging wildflowers. When you see thick mats of pine straw and large cones, you look up to see clumps of longleaf pine. On stretches of the Pinhoti south of this, closer to the FS 500 trailhead, longleaf predominates.

This ridge hiking continues through several false starts until finally the trail begins a steep descent toward the Lower Shoal Shelter. Here, two mountain streams converge, one of them dropping down a small waterfall. It's a serene place to sleep, listening to the flow of the water. There's a picnic table here too.

The hike out is fairly steep, with 250 feet of elevation gain in a little more than half a mile, but you get another taste of great views, and your car should be waiting when you reach FS 531.

Directions

Take I-20 East toward Atlanta and take Exit 191 (US 431/US 78). At the end of the ramp, take a left (north), headed toward US 78. Go half a mile and turn right (east), onto US 78. Go 5.6 miles and take a left onto CR 500/Scenic Drive. At the next intersection, continue straight across Skyway Motorway to unpaved FS 500. Cross train tracks and proceed 2.5 miles to the intersection with FS 531. Take a left onto 531 and proceed 0.8 mile to the spot where the Pinhoti crosses the road. Drop one car here on the shoulder, making sure not to block the road. Continue up FS 531 for 2.8 miles and locate the trailhead near Highrock Lake. Park off the road, away from low spots and creek and trail crossings. If it's raining or likely to rain heavily, don't park here.

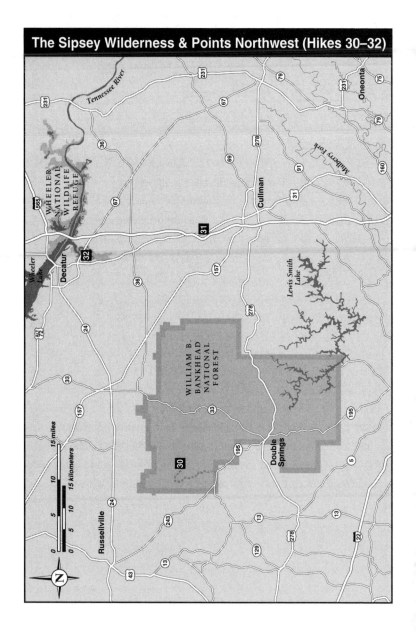

The Sipsey Wilderness & Points Northwest (Hikes 30–32)

The Sipsey Wilderness & Points Northwest

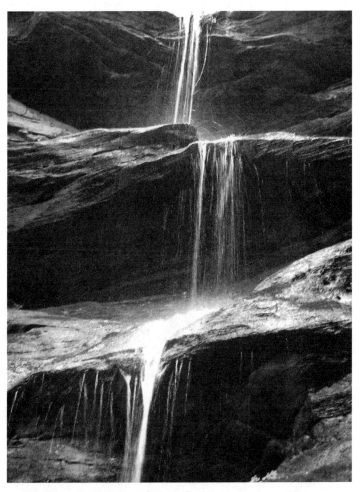

A WATERFALL DROPS DOWN CANYON WALLS IN THE SIPSEY WILDERNESS.
(See Hike 30.)

Sipsey Wilderness & Points Northwest Overview

WHEN YOU ASK PEOPLE TO NAME their favorite hiking destination in Alabama, the Sipsey Wilderness in the Bankhead National Forest is the most common answer. This is despite the fact that the Sipsey takes some extra effort to get to.

North and west of Birmingham, you find a different terrain and forest type. Instead of long-running ridges and wide valleys, the land is rumpled with ups and downs. Common features include deep hollows, coves, and canyons that have been cut into the countryside by streams and rivers.

These refuges often feature waterfalls and a cool, shady microclimate where you can find hemlock trees, massive beech trees, giant-leafed deciduous magnolias, and mossy boulders.

The best showcase for this *Land Before Time* landscape is the Sipsey Wilderness. Deep in the area are pockets of primeval forest

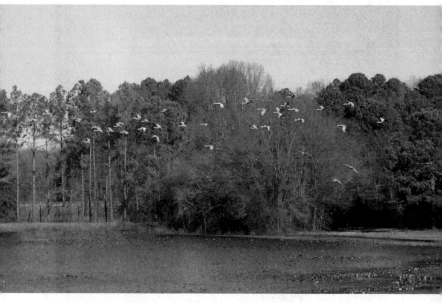

A FLOCK OF SANDHILL CRANES GLIDES ABOVE DUCKS AND OTHER WATERFOWL FEEDING IN CRABTREE SLOUGH, IN THE WHEELER NATIONAL WILDLIFE REFUGE. *(See Hike 32.)*

that have never been cut for timber. These remnant old-growth forests stand today as an enduring tribute to a dedicated band of conservationists, including Mary Ivy Burks of Birmingham, a founder of the Alabama Environmental Council.

Through the 1960s, the federal government considered wilderness to be something found way out in the West. It took years of lobbying, but finally supporters of the Eastern Wilderness Movement, including Burks, convinced Congress that special pockets of wilderness in the East deserved long-term protection too.

The Sipsey Wilderness, created in 1975 and expanded in 1988, was among the first designated wilderness areas east of the Mississippi River. At 24,922 acres, the Sipsey is one of the larger wilderness areas in the eastern United States.

The **Big Tree Loop** hike, on page 241, takes you into the heart of the wilderness to the tallest tree in Alabama, a 150-foot-tall tulip poplar estimated to be 500 years old. It also features a beautiful amble along the clear-running, boulder-strewn course of the Sipsey Fork of the Black Warrior River.

For a much easier introduction to the Sipsey, try an out-and-back hike on the **Borden Creek Trail** (Forest Service Road 200) from the Sipsey River Recreational Area to the Borden Creek Trailhead. Parking for the recreational area is on Cranal Road (FS 4 or County Road 60).

For easy access to a similar but less remote landscape, try **Hurricane Creek Park,** near Cullman (Hike 31, page 249).

Also described in this section is a pilgrimage to the **Wheeler National Wildlife Refuge,** on the banks of the Tennessee River. The peak time to go is in January, when you're guaranteed to see sandhill cranes. If you're lucky, you'll also see one of the rarest and most majestic birds alive, the whooping crane. Along with the viewing areas adjacent to the visitor center, you can try out several other hiking options. In the winter, the roads through the refuge are closed to traffic, so you can ride a bike for miles.

Note: The Sipsey Wilderness has seen an invasion of feral hogs in recent years. It's doubtful that you'll see a hog, especially during the day, but you will see where they've rooted the ground, particularly under acorn-producing oak trees. This is not just a gentle upturning of leaves but something closer to plowing. Feral hogs will also create wallows in wetlands and creeks, in some cases destroying stream banks or trails. While these animals are shy and not generally a threat to humans, you'll want to think twice about bringing a dog. The pigs carry a virus known as pseudorabies—humans aren't susceptible, but for dogs it's a killer, producing symptoms that mimic the derangement of the rabies virus. If you do bring your pet, keep him on a leash and out of the hog wallows, where standing water might be contaminated with the virus.

Other Area Attractions

AVE MARIA GROTTO A classic Alabama roadside attraction, Ave Maria Grotto is on the grounds of the St. Bernard Abbey in Cullman. Over the course of 40 years, Benedictine monk Joseph Zoettl recreated, in folk-art miniature, holy sites from around the world. The weathered pastiche of concrete, colored glass, marbles, cold-cream jars, scraps of marble, broken bathroom tile, and costume jewelry covers 3 acres. Open daily, 9 a.m.–5 p.m.; admission is $7 for adults, $5 for seniors and AAA members, and $4.50 for kids ages 6–12. 1600 St. Bernard Dr. SE, Cullman; 256-734-4110, **avemariagrotto.com.**

BIG BOB GIBSON BAR-B-Q After birding, try some world-famous barbecue from Big Bob's. Open daily, 9:30 a.m.–8:15 p.m. 1715 Sixth Ave. SE (US 31), Decatur; 256-350-6969, **bigbobgibson.com.**

JESSE OWENS MEMORIAL PARK A public park with ball fields, basketball courts, picnic pavilions, and playgrounds. A museum and a replica of Owens's childhood home on the grounds tell the inspiring story of the Alabama native who won four gold medals at the 1936 Berlin Olympics. Museum and home replica open Monday–Saturday, 10 a.m.–4 p.m., and Sunday, 1–4 p.m.; free admission. The park is accessible anytime. 7019 County Rd. 203, Danville; 256-974-3636, **jesseowensmemorialpark.com.**

30

Big Tree Loop

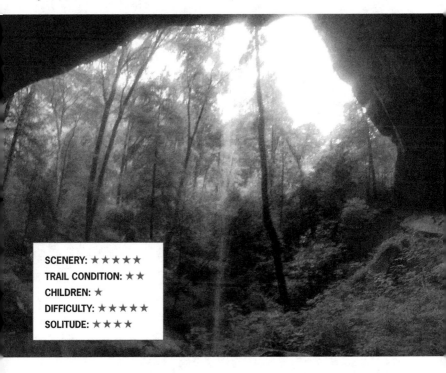

SCENERY: ★ ★ ★ ★ ★
TRAIL CONDITION: ★ ★
CHILDREN: ★
DIFFICULTY: ★ ★ ★ ★ ★
SOLITUDE: ★ ★ ★ ★

GPS TRAILHEAD COORDINATES: N34° 20.454' W87° 28.230'

DISTANCE & CONFIGURATION: 10.8-mile loop—but see below regarding distance

HIKING TIME: 7 hours

HIGHLIGHTS: Bee Branch Falls, Alabama's largest tree, cool hemlock canyons, mossy boulders and rocky overhangs, and the clear waters of the Sipsey Fork

ELEVATION: 620' at the start; 980' at the high point; 574' at the low point

ACCESS: The trails of the Sipsey Wilderness are free and always open; camping allowed.

MAPS: *Sipsey Wilderness & Black Warrior Wildlife Management Area of the William B. Bankhead National Forest,* by Carto-Craft of Birmingham; USGS *Bee Branch, AL*

FACILITIES: None

WHEELCHAIR ACCESS: None

COMMENTS: Park before you reach the bridge over the creek. Cross the metal bridge to the trailhead. Different sources have measured the distance at anywhere from 10.8 miles to more than 12 miles—be prepared to err on the side of longer.

CONTACTS: US Forest Service, Bankhead Ranger District, 205-489-5111, **www.fs.usda .gov/alabama;** Sipsey River Hiking Club, **sipseywilderness.org**

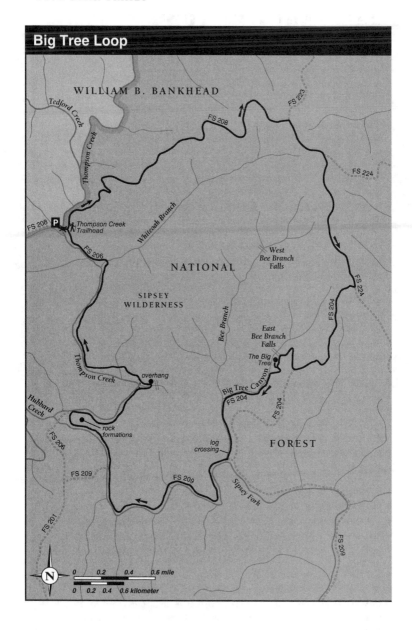

Big Tree Loop

WILLIAM B. BANKHEAD

Tedford Creek

Thompson Creek

FS 208

FS 223

FS 224

FS 208

P Thompson Creek Trailhead

FS 206

Whiteoak Branch

West Bee Branch Falls

FS 224

NATIONAL

SIPSEY WILDERNESS

FS 204

Bee Branch

East Bee Branch Falls

The Big Tree

Thompson Creek

overhang

Big Tree Canyon

FS 204

FS 204

Hubbard Creek

rock formations

log crossing

FOREST

FS 206

FS 209

FS 209

FS 201

Sipsey Fork

FS 209

N

0   0.2   0.4   0.6 mile

0   0.2   0.4   0.6 kilometer

Overview

This 10.8-mile loop from Thompson Creek Trailhead in the northwest portion of the Sipsey Wilderness features well-known landmarks of the wilderness, including Bee Branch Falls, rock formations and river rapids along the Sipsey Fork, and the "Big Tree," a towering yellow poplar reputed to be Alabama's tallest tree.

This is a full-day hump that explores varied terrain and forest types. It has some elevation gain and creek crossings. Some trail sections are among the most popular in the wilderness, and numerous campsites line the path. This loop proceeds clockwise from the Thompson Creek Trailhead up Forest Service Road 208 (Northwest Road) to FS 224 (Bunyan Hill) to FS 204 (Bee Ridge) to FS 209 (Sipsey River) to FS 206 (Thompson Creek).

Route Details

An expedition in the Sipsey Wilderness to the Big Tree is something of a rite of passage for Alabama hikers. On our expedition, we were miles deep in the wilderness, and yet we ran into two other parties wandering East Bee Branch Canyon, trying to pin down the exact location of the Big Tree, a 150-foot-tall yellow poplar that the Forest Service estimates to be 500 years old.

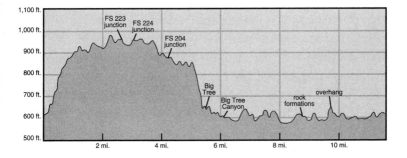

You'd think a tree like that would be impossible to miss, but this *is* a wilderness, and there aren't large directional signposts. But you'll know it when you see it. It stands alone, bulging in girth, its top stretching skyward seemingly beyond sight. It's the centerpiece of a wilderness cathedral, cupped by the enclosing cliffs at the far end of East Bee Branch Canyon and within sight of two high, single-stream waterfalls (at least in wet weather).

But I have to admit that I didn't find it the first three times I tried.

And that was OK, because the real reward of the quest for the Big Tree is the journey itself, through old-growth forest that seems both timeless and utterly organically young and alive. Tiny frogs hop. Lizards scamper. Trees grip moss-covered boulders with roots that look like octopus legs. The river burbles and courses. The hawk cries.

Though there are more direct routes to the Big Tree, this route takes you through varied terrain and past many Sipsey Wilderness landmarks. As a general outline, this loop hike climbs to a plateau and travels along the ridge before descending East Bee Branch Canyon to the Sipsey River, which you will then follow back upstream to its junction with Thompson Creek. The trail then meanders up Thompson Creek back to the trailhead and parking lot.

Expect a 2-hour drive from the Birmingham city center to the Thompson Creek Trailhead, at the dead end of FS 208. Then expect a full day of hiking.

We started at 10 a.m., kept a pretty steady pace without a lot of resting, and returned at 5 p.m. The digital cartography for this book yielded a distance of 10.8 miles, but the odometer on my GPS unit indicated we'd been more than 12 miles . . . and it felt like it.

Across a metal bridge from the parking area is a kiosk. Facing it, take note of the FS 206 trail to your right—that's how you'll make your return. To begin our hike, take FS 208 to the left (northeast), up what used to be a county road. FS 208 is designated as path for horseback riding, which means it's wider than a footpath. Downed trees tend to get cleared, which is a bonus.

You'll be walking through a forest that is predominantly hard-wood with a sprinkling of pines of various species. Almost immediately you notice that trees are larger here. Most Alabama forests, even on public lands, have been cut in the relatively recent past, but some areas of the wilderness, thanks to its general inaccessibility, may never have been logged. As you climb, you can see nearby ridges and get a sense of the surrounding topography, which amounts to an old mountain plateau that has become crosscut by innumerable narrow canyons carved by small creeks.

Thanks to the mature canopy of trees, the forest doesn't have that tangle of undergrowth you see elsewhere. When a deer became aware of our presence and we of hers, we were treated to a long show of her graceful and not particularly hurried retreat down the draw deeper into the wilderness.

That was not the only evidence of wildlife we saw. Shortly thereafter, we began to see disturbances in the leaf litter along the edges of the road, particularly under large oaks. In places it almost looked as if machinery had been through, and on a portion of trail higher on the ridge, the roughed-up ground included the trail itself, creating muddy wallows that were a challenge to navigate.

This is the work of an overgrown population of feral hogs that lives in the wilderness. They aren't a threat to humans, and they stay hidden during the day, but they are a menace to the forest ecosystem, plowing through patches of precious plants and tearing up the banks of creeks. They are also a danger to dogs. (See the area overview, pages 239–240, for more information.)

At the top of the ridge, you'll intersect FS 223 (Gum Pond Trail or County Road 7). Continue on FS 208 to the right (southeast). Not long thereafter, the trail splits, and again you bear right (south), this time on FS 224 (Bunyan Hill Trail). Just short of 4 miles into the hike, you'll see a trail sign offering an option to go to the right on FS 204 (Bee Ridge Trail). Take FS 204 to begin your descent toward Bee Branch Canyon.

Beginning on this section and continuing throughout the rest of the hike, you'll frequently see well-used campsites along the trail.

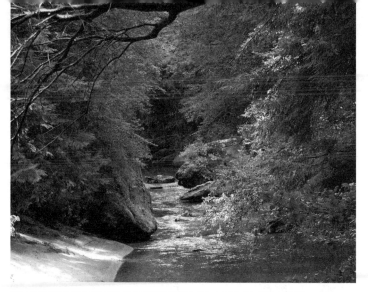

THE SIPSEY FORK OF THE BLACK WARRIOR RIVER MAKES ITS WAY THROUGH A COURSE OF BOULDERS.

Individual sites should not host more than 10 people, and campers are encouraged to camp off the trail itself. Though it would seem to go without saying, pack out any trash you bring in. Unfortunately, not everyone has gotten that message.

A short distance downhill, FS 204 splits. A trail marker is carved into the tree. Take the spur to the right, known as 204A, the East Bee Branch Canyon Trail. If you need a clue and there has been decent rain of late, listen carefully and you'll hear the water of East Bee Branch. Hike in that direction. As you descend into the canyon, you'll start to see rhododendron and hemlock. These plants are typically found farther north in cooler climates but the narrow canyons of the Sipsey and the Bankhead stay cooler. They are shady and moist, and they create a refuge for these plants, which were much more common in Alabama during the last Ice Age. That lost-world feeling grows as you go deeper into the canyon.

You'll see trail spurs descend steeply toward the branch and to East Bee Branch Falls, a sublime sight. This is the highest set of falls in the Bankhead but by no means the largest or widest. Its narrowness is essential to its charm, its fountain springing from the dry upland woods and falling into a mossy grotto far below. Be very careful near the edge. It's a very long way down, and there is nothing between you and the edge.

From this high vantage point you can look down the canyon and see tremendous oaks, poplars, and hemlocks.

After viewing the falls, trace your way back to the trail and continue until you reach a junction where the trail descends steeply to the right, into the canyon and in the direction of the branch. Take care making the descent. You'll reach an unmarked trail junction. Go right, toward the base of the falls—the Big Tree will appear in the foreground with East Bee Branch Falls in the background.

Take some time to savor this special place. Then, if you like, explore the area behind Bee Branch Falls or the second waterfall nearby, but be careful. The rocks are slippery and the ground muddy.

When you're ready to leave, retrace your footsteps to the trail junction where you descended and then proceed along the trail that parallels East Bee Branch on its southeast side.

From the time you leave the falls until you reach the river, the trail will be somewhat difficult to trace. Hikers have created various spurs to scenic spots. Further, the tornadoes of 2011 ripped through the wilderness and left numerous fallen trees, around which hikers have improvised paths. You'll pass through mazes of mossy boulders along the branch. On our visit during a wet summer, the trail featured a multitude of mushrooms of various shapes and sizes. We spotted frogs along this stretch and salamanders tucked up in the crevices of the rocks.

East Bee Branch is joined by West Bee Branch, and the two make their way to the Sipsey Fork. At the river, FS 204A intersects FS 209, which follows the river. Crossing Bee Branch to head upstream on FS 209 can be a challenge.

We were there after a period of rain and ended up getting bogged down in mud. About 100 feet upstream from the junction with the Sipsey, a downed tree lies across the branch. You can cross here if you have good balance.

Once across, you'll be hiking along the Sipsey Fork, Alabama's only federally designated Wild and Scenic River. The river is variable in character along its course and dependent on recent rainfall. When we hiked it, the river was clear blue and green, with slow-moving pools broken by rapids and falls threaded through rock formations. Tremendous boulders line the bank, interspersed with sandy banks, providing several spots to stop and take in the scenery.

We continued on the same side of the river until we met the junction with FS 206 at Thompson Creek. This final leg back to the parking lot is a tad disorienting at points, as it temporarily jogs to the west away from Thompson Creek, but keep the faith and follow the FS 206 trail signs back to the trailhead.

Official trail maps show Trails 209 and 206 making stream crossings. Ignore them. Stay on the right-hand bank of both the Sipsey Fork and Thompson Creek, headed upstream.

Nearby Attractions

On your way out, if you didn't take a dip in the Sipsey, you can stop at **Kinlock Falls,** a well-known swimming hole and natural rock slide. It's on FS 210 (Kinlock Road or CR 2) on your way out, shortly after a historical marker for Kinlock Springs. Several small pulloff parking spots are arranged around a sharp bend in the road; otherwise, the site is poorly marked. The falls are on Hubbard Creek.

Directions

Take I-65 North to Exit 308. Head left (west) on US 278 for 37 miles to Double Springs. Just as you enter Double Springs, turn right (north) onto AL 33. After 12.5 miles, turn left (west) onto Cranal Road (CR 6), which soon becomes CR 60. The Sipsey River Recreation Area and several other trailheads are along this road. Cranal Road dead-ends into Kinlock Road (FS 210). Take a right and drive on Kinlock 6.2 miles. Along the way, it turns into a dirt road. You'll intersect FS 203, bear right, and, 0.4 mile later, take a right onto FS 208 (Northwest Road or CR 3). Four miles later the road ends, with gravel parking available just before a metal bridge that is closed to vehicular traffic.

31

Hurricane Creek Park

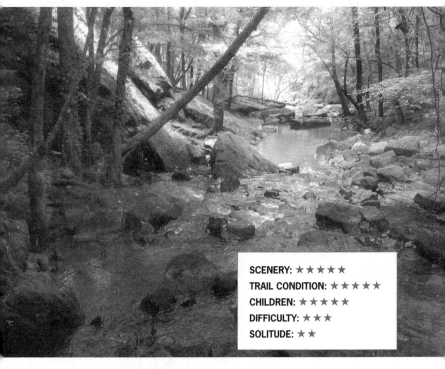

SCENERY: ★ ★ ★ ★ ★
TRAIL CONDITION: ★ ★ ★ ★ ★
CHILDREN: ★ ★ ★ ★ ★
DIFFICULTY: ★ ★ ★
SOLITUDE: ★ ★

GPS TRAILHEAD COORDINATES: N34° 17.206' W86° 53.676'

DISTANCE & CONFIGURATION: Double loop of about 2 miles

HIKING TIME: 3 hours, with time for lunch

HIGHLIGHTS: Numerous waterfalls and rock formations, including the cavelike Twilight Tunnel; clear water and large boulders on Hurricane Creek; diverse old-growth flora and fauna

ELEVATION: 775' at the start and at the natural bridge; 610' at the low point

ACCESS: Open Friday, noon–sunset; Saturday and Sunday, 9 a.m.–sunset; Closed Monday–Thursday. Admission is $3 for adults, $2.50 for children age 17 and under; admission for groups of 10 or more is $2/person; cash only.

MAPS: Trail map available at park headquarters

FACILITIES: Restrooms and concessions at headquarters; rock-climbing gear and climbing walls; picnic areas by the creek

WHEELCHAIR ACCESS: None

COMMENTS: Hurricane Creek is also known as the William "Buddy" Rodgers Natural Area, in memory of the park's founder.

CONTACT: 256-734-2125, **hurricanecreek.homestead.com**

Hurricane Creek Park

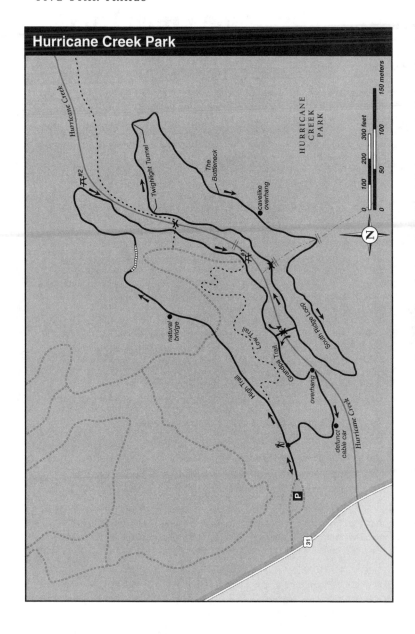

Overview

Right off US 31 north of Cullman, this 500-foot-deep canyon preserve offers quick, convenient access to a woodland wonderland of rain-fed waterfalls, rock formations, and old-growth flora and fauna. You can take a short, steep scenic hike to the creek at the bottom of the canyon or wander loops that explore the canyon walls. For the adventurous and non-claustrophobic, don't miss Twilight Tunnel or The Bottleneck on the South Ridge Loop. Guided rock-climbing adventures are offered on Saturdays.

Route Details

Hurricane Creek Park originally opened in 1961 as a private attraction by William "Buddy" Rodgers. A Decatur native, Rodgers (who died in 2008) went off to World War II and became a decorated fighter pilot, flying P-47 Thunderbolts in the European theater. Read more about his adventures on the website or when you visit the park.

Back home, he was flying over northern Cullman County as part of a mapping project when, from the air, he spotted this canyon atop Lacon Mountain. He went back and explored it on the ground, persuaded the owners to sell, and, after cutting trails and building bridges, opened the park for hiking and picnicking. Rodgers served as its beloved host for 40 years.

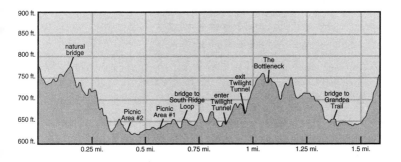

In 2003, he donated the 67-acre property to the state of Alabama. The Cullman City Parks and Recreation Department has restored and improved the facilities and trails and now maintains and operates the park. Especially well developed is Hurricane Creek's rock-climbing program, which includes a well-stocked pro shop and climbing walls at park headquarters. Introductory rock-climbing expeditions are offered every Saturday.

Trail maps are available in the park office. The trails are all well marked, though owing to years of use they have many unsanctioned offshoots. For conservation's sake, try to stay on the trail. The newer green-and-white trail signs are the ones you want to follow.

Depending on your inclination, you can hike short or long, but what you can't avoid is steep.

It's a mildly challenging walk up and down, and there are some edges you'll want to avoid falling off of. Stick to the trail and keep your eye on the kids, and you'll be fine.

Since we had the whole day available and didn't want to miss any of the attractions, we chose to take the High Trail, which winds along the north rim of the canyon; cross the creek at the bottom of the canyon; and hike the South Ridge Loop, up the other ridge and through the Twilight Tunnel before returning to the picnic areas along the creek. We ate, swam, and took a shorter, steeper path up Heaven's Staircase back to the park headquarters. All that took about 3.5 hours.

To follow that route, start at the trailhead at the rear of the headquarters, and proceed straight rather than taking the immediate option to descend toward the creek and Twilight Tunnel. Bear in mind that Twilight Tunnel is on the South Ridge Loop. We'll get to that later.

Shortly after you begin, you cross a narrow wooden bridge. If you haven't already, start looking at the flora, which transitions from the typical Alabama landscape to a primeval world: cowcumber magnolias, with their tremendous broad leaves, rise overhead. The cowcumber is a deciduous cousin of the more common evergreen magnolia. You'll also see a generous supply of oakleaf hydrangea and evergreen mountain laurel along the path.

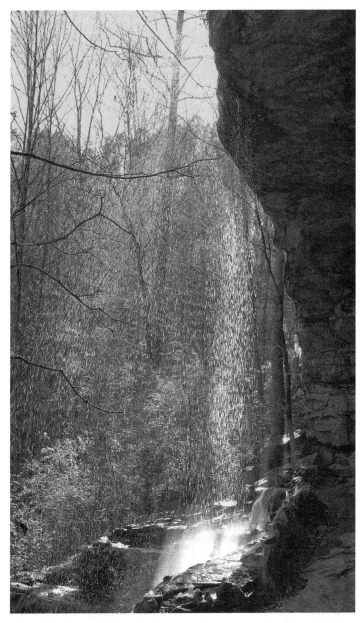

A WET-WEATHER WATERFALL DROPS FROM THE CLIFFS AT HURRICANE CREEK PARK.

After crossing a maintenance road that heads steeply downhill, you'll see, on your left, the first unusual rock formation, a natural bridge of stone. Stop to explore. The trail system also offers benches at good spots for contemplating the scenery and sounds.

From this point on, you'll be navigating through rock formations, under overhangs, and along ledges. As the canyon deepens, it becomes more moist and more deeply shaded. Mosses and ferns abound. Small creeks descend the ridges to feed Hurricane Creek at the base of the canyon, forming delicate waterfalls along their course.

Most of these dry up in the heat of the summer, but in the cooler months, as many as 15 can be found throughout the length of the trail system.

After winding down the mountainside, you reach Hurricane Creek and Picnic Area #2. Look for a picnic table atop a large boulder here; other spots farther downstream offer more-secluded dining and reflection.

To keep hiking, proceed upstream toward Picnic Area #1, situated at a point in the creek where a small man-made rock dam forms an upper and lower pool and a waterfall. We returned to this spot for our picnic and for some swimming. Large boulders on the creek banks look like great jumping points, but the creek is rather shallow. Take care.

We pressed on, following the signs to Twilight Tunnel. Upstream from Picnic Area #1, a two-bridge system crosses from the north side of the creek to the south. On the opposite bank, you hike up a bit and then take a left onto the loop toward Twilight Tunnel, heading back downstream. After a short distance, you reach the tunnel, a tall, narrow crack in a conglomeration of tremendous boulders.

As you proceed inside, it gets progressively darker and narrower until, at one point, it's too dark to see anything. A few steps later, light peeks through another opening above. Continue carefully, through and over unseen obstacles. Watch your footing. At the far end, you climb out of the tunnel and find yourself on a tall boulder overlooking the canyon.

Continue uphill to rejoin the loop trail, which bypasses the tunnel. Signs here give you a choice of returning to the picnic area or continuing on the South Ridge Loop, which is about 1 mile long. We continued on the loop. Some of the biggest old-growth trees are found farther along. The south ridge takes some mild exertion but pays off. There's The Bottleneck, a narrow squeeze through boulders. Had I shed my backpack and camera, I could have squeezed through, but the twinge of panic I felt in the constriction was enough for me. I backed out and took the bypass.

Farther up the ridge, a deep, cavelike overhang offers chances to explore, plus creeks, waterfalls, and views.

All too soon, you've completed the loop. You have a choice of how to get back to the park office: If you return to Picnic Area #1, you can make a steep but enjoyable ascent of stairs built into the rocks—a course labeled Heaven's Staircase, which leads you on what's referred to on the park map as the Low Trail. Or you can proceed upstream on the creek on the Grandpa Trail, making a more gradual ascent. In wet weather, that route offers another tall waterfall and a peek at the defunct cable car that used to ferry people up from the base of the canyon.

Nearby Attractions

Cullman is also home to **Ave Maria Grotto,** a hillside landscape of sculptures on the grounds of St. Bernard Abbey. See page 240 for more information.

Directions

Take I-65 to Exit 318 (Lacon/Vinemont). Turn right (south) onto US 31 and proceed about 1 mile. Look for signs for Hurricane Creek Park, which is on the left at the bottom of a hill. US 31 in this stretch has unusual concrete medians; don't miss the gap in the median that allows you to turn into the parking lot.

32

Wheeler National Wildlife Refuge

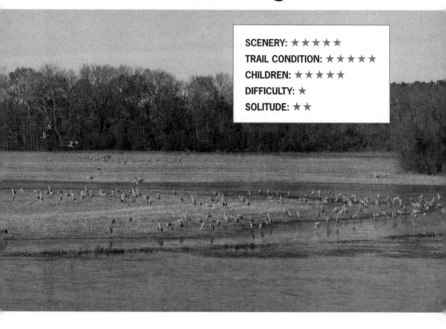

SCENERY: ★ ★ ★ ★
TRAIL CONDITION: ★ ★ ★ ★ ★
CHILDREN: ★ ★ ★ ★
DIFFICULTY: ★
SOLITUDE: ★ ★

GPS TRAILHEAD COORDINATES: N34° 32.843' W86° 57.064'

DISTANCE & CONFIGURATION: 1 mile

HIKING TIME: Less than an hour

HIGHLIGHTS: A birder's paradise on the banks of the Tennessee River: Winter in the refuge offers a chance to see whooping cranes, one of the world's most magnificent and most endangered birds, along with thousands of sandhill cranes, ducks, geese, and other waterfowl.

ACCESS: Visitor Center open October–February, 9 a.m.–5 p.m., and March–September, 9 a.m.–4 p.m.; closed July 4, Thanksgiving Day, and December 25

ELEVATION: Very little change, from 559' to 564'

MAPS: Available at the Visitor Center and at the website below

FACILITIES: Visitor center, picnic tables

WHEELCHAIR ACCESS: Yes

COMMENTS: In addition to birding and hiking, the refuge offers hunting and fishing, boating, and even bicycling on more than 100 miles of roads that are closed to vehicular traffic during the winter.

CONTACT: Wheeler National Wildlife Refuge, 256-353-7243, **fws.gov/wheeler**

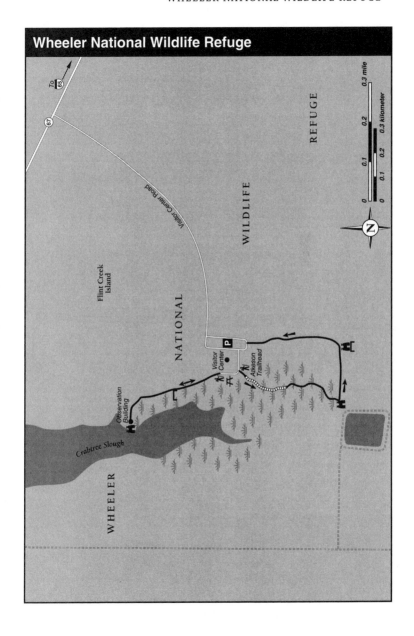

Wheeler National Wildlife Refuge

Overview

The hike described is short but likely to be very rewarding in the right season. A short walk from the Visitor Center is a specially constructed observation building, where you have a good chance of seeing the cranes that winter here on the banks of the Tennessee River.

Route Details

I pulled up to the gates of Wheeler National Wildlife Refuge at 9 a.m. on a January morning, just before the gates to the Visitor Center road were to open. Above the fields of stubble that lay beyond the gate, the blue skies were filled with sandhill cranes. With wingspans exceeding 6 feet, the cranes came in groups, flying in formation from every direction, flapping and gliding and honking to one another in continuous conversation as they came.

I went scrambling for my camera, thinking I had arrived at a highly unusual moment that I urgently needed to capture. It turned out to be just the beginning of a morning of ongoing wonder.

The hike I'm going to describe is barely a mile. If you really want to stretch your legs, Wheeler offers several other options. The Flint Creek Trail is a pleasant walk in hardwood bottom forest along the Tennessee River, just across the highway from the visitor center. There are also more than 100 miles of roads that are closed to cars during the winter but are open to walkers and bicyclers.

What you can't miss are the short, scenic, wheelchair-accessible walks around the visitor center. Beginning around Thanksgiving, peaking in January, and tapering after that, Wheeler offers one of the state's great natural spectacles.

I say "natural," but there's some human influence at work here. Wheeler National Wildlife Refuge was created as something of an afterthought to the Tennessee Valley Authority's damming and harnessing of the Tennessee River. A buffer of land along the new reservoir was set aside as a breeding ground for migratory birds and other wildlife in 1938 by President Franklin D. Roosevelt. Much of the 3,500-acre refuge is planted annually by local farmers who lease the land and, as part of the arrangement, leave a portion of their crop in the field for the birds to eat.

In recent years, about 75,000 ducks and 2,000 geese have wintered in the refuge. Sandhill cranes, once rare, have exploded in number, with winter populations reaching 12,000 or more. In recent years, sandhills have been joined by whooping cranes. In the late 1930s, whooping cranes had been hunted nearly to extinction, with fewer than 20 of the birds surviving. An intensive international effort has brought the population up to about 600 wild birds. Starting in 2006 with a single pair, Wheeler's delegation of whooping cranes was about a dozen strong in 2014. The refuge now hosts a festival of the cranes in January, when populations are at their peak.

The sight I saw that Saturday morning was the cranes heading in for breakfast at Crabtree Slough, just beyond the observation building adjacent to the visitor center. The cranes spend the night dispersed along the river in the shallow mudflats, where they are safe from creeping coyotes. As the sun gets higher, they return en masse to their feeding grounds.

To see them up close, your first stop is the Visitor Center itself. Here, you can get maps and directions and take in the explanatory exhibits and a film about the refuge's history and wildlife.

Behind the Visitor Center are two trails. To the left (south) is the Atkeson Trail, and to the north is the Wildlife Observation Trail, leading out to the Observation Building. First let's take the Atkeson Trail, a loop of close to half a mile. Named after Tom Atkeson, a longtime manager of the refuge, the trail begins with an elevated boardwalk through a cypress swamp. When I was there, the towering trees were bare and beautiful, their wide-based trunks rising from the ice that topped the brown-bottomed swamp. Leaving the boardwalk, the trail continues in a wooded area with a few winding trail options that cut back along the high ground beside other wetlands. I continued north to the far end of the wooded area, arriving at the edge of an open field, where a sign and gate instruct you to stop. In the distance, I spotted a large congregation

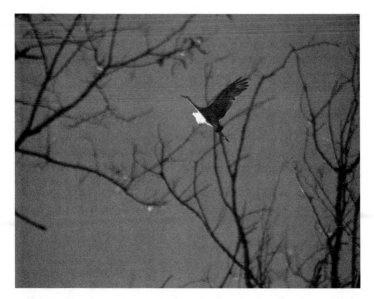

SANDHILL CRANES GATHER BY THE THOUSANDS AT WHEELER NATIONAL WILDLIFE REFUGE.

of sandhills plus two pairs of whooping cranes, which stood out stark white in contrast with their gray-feathered companions. Both cranes sport a red crown on the top of their head.

As I walked back toward the visitor center on the trails tracing the perimeter of the forest, I looked out into adjacent fields from the cover of the trees. Several cranes flew low overhead. The trek back also offers some interesting wandering possibilities through a glade of giant bamboo. It's an invasive species, but it does make for an interesting landscape.

Return to the rear of the visitor center. The Wildlife Observation Trail heads north through another tree-sheltered corridor about 200 yards to the Observation Building. Here, through the one-way glass, you can see out over a marsh where thousands of ducks, geese, and sandhill cranes congregate. With all the takeoffs and landings going on, the scene looked like a very busy airport. The sandhills seemed to be able to hover in the air on approach. They jumped and danced with one another. The whooping cranes, white with black highlights on their wings, were regal but didn't seem to mind sharing the marsh. A variety of ducks, mallards, teals, and wood ducks floated on the open water.

The two-story building has a speaker system and directional microphones that allow visitors to hear the sounds on the pond. Spotting scopes help you see the birds up close. If you've ever wanted to feel like you were on the set of a National Geographic special, here's your chance. It's a short drive up the interstate.

Nearby Attractions

Barbecue fans know **Big Bob Gibson's** (see page 240) in Decatur, not far from the refuge. When you return to AL 67, instead of heading south back toward the interstate, head north to reach US 31. Take a right, going north on US 31; the landmark restaurant will be on your left.

If the limited hiking at the refuge hasn't satisfied you, Cullman's **Hurricane Creek Park** (Hike 31, page 249) is on your way back, at Exit 318 off I-65.

Directions

Take I-65 North to Exit 334 (Decatur/Priceville). At the end of the exit ramp, take a left onto AL 67. Travel 2.8 miles northwest to the visitor center entrance road, on the left.

Little River Canyon & Points Northeast (Hikes 33–35)

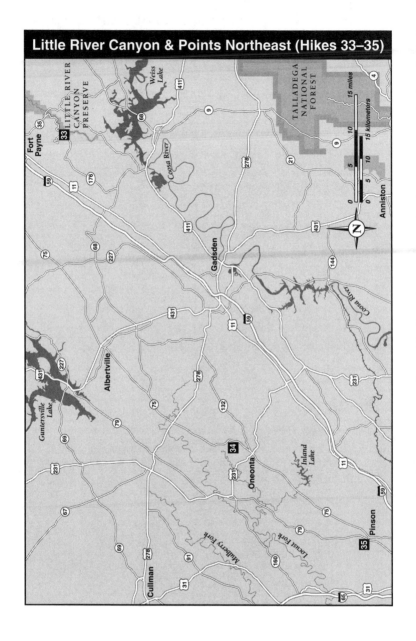

Little River Canyon
& Points Northeast

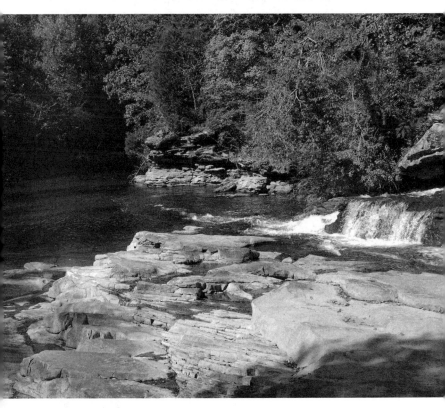

TURKEY CREEK FALLS HAS LONG BEEN A GATHERING PLACE AND
SWIMMING HOLE IN NORTHEAST JEFFERSON COUNTY. *(See Hike 35.)*

Little River Canyon & Points Northeast Overview

DRIVE NORTHEAST FROM BIRMINGHAM and you're headed into the Cumberland Plateau region, a terrain of steep-sided but flat-topped mountains, the most prominent being Sand and Lookout Mountains.

The hikes in this section start at the southern edge of these plateaus, at **Turkey Creek Nature Preserve** in Pinson. Farther north in Blount County, near Oneonta, is **Palisades Park,** and north and east of there, atop Lookout Mountain, is **Little River Canyon.**

At Palisades Park, you get to stand atop sandstone cliffs and look out over the edge of one of these plateaus for a dramatic view. At Little River Canyon, you'll get equally dramatic views, but this time from the cliffs overlooking a gash cut into the Lookout Mountain plateau by Little River. Both are great spots to view fall colors.

All three of these hikes offer a beat-the-heat option. **Turkey Creek Falls** at the preserve is a classic swimming hole. You can dip your toes in the **Locust Fork of the Black Warrior River** at Swann Bridge on the way home from Palisades Park. And Little River Canyon offers multiple swimming holes along the course of the river.

Other Area Attractions

LOOKOUT MOUNTAIN

DeSOTO STATE PARK On the Lookout Mountain Plateau, north of Little River Canyon, is DeSoto State Park, which is lovely in and of itself but which also provides a convenient base of operations for exploring Little River Canyon and the rest of the plateau. Highlights include **DeSoto Falls,** where the Little River makes a dramatic 104-foot drop into the gorge. 13903 County Road 89, Fort Payne; 800-568-8840; **alapark.com/desotoresort.**

FORT PAYNE This area is significant in Cherokee Indian history. Wills Town, a Presbyterian mission to the Cherokees, was founded in 1816. Sequoyah, inventor of the Cherokee alphabet, lived there for a time. During the forced removal of the Cherokees from the South in the 1830s, Fort Payne was a gathering and departure point for the

Trail of Tears, the grueling relocation march to Oklahoma. On a happier and more recent note, the **Alabama Fan Club and Museum** is located at 101 Glenn Blvd. SW; 256-845-1646, **thealabamaband.com.**

NOCCALULA FALLS PARK Just north of Gadsden and accessible from Exit 188 off I-59, a city park features a 90-foot-tall waterfall on Black Creek. Look for a statue on the cliffs of a Cherokee Indian maiden who supposedly jumped to her death in the falls rather than go through with an arranged marriage. Along with the long-standing route to the base of the falls, new trails have been added to the park by the city of Gadsden.

Also consider a visit to **Mentone** (**mentonealabama.gov**), a charming mountain town and summer-camp central, north of DeSoto State Park.

SAND MOUNTAIN

BUCK'S POCKET STATE PARK Small but scenic state park in a narrow gorge cut into Sand Mountain by South Sauty Creek. Great views from the bluffs above the gorge, plus hiking and camping. 393 County Rd. 174, Grove Oak; 256-659-2000, **alapark.com/buckspocket.**

LAKE GUNTERSVILLE STATE PARK The park lodge is perched high on a bluff overlooking the 69,000-acre Guntersville Reservoir. Attractions include hiking trails and bald-eagle viewing in winter. 7966 AL Hwy. 227, Guntersville; 256-571-5444, **alapark.com/lakeguntersville.**

Even farther off the beaten path is **High Falls** (**seehighfalls.com**). Off AL 75, this 300-foot-wide, 35-foot-tall waterfall is formed by Town Creek. Worth the diversion.

Outfitters

ONE WORLD ADVENTURE COMPANY Offers guided treks for hiking, canoeing, rock climbing, and camping in Mentone; 256-634-8370, **oneworldadventureco.com.**

TRUE ADVENTURE SPORTS Outdoor recreational outfitters for rock climbing, rappelling, zip-lining, camping, and paddling; guided trips and lessons. 13102 AL Hwy. 176, Fort Payne; 256-997-9577, **trueadventuresports.com.**

33

Little River Canyon National Preserve:
Eberhart Trail

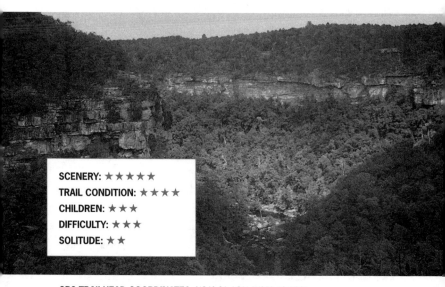

SCENERY: ★ ★ ★ ★ ★
TRAIL CONDITION: ★ ★ ★ ★
CHILDREN: ★ ★ ★
DIFFICULTY: ★ ★ ★
SOLITUDE: ★ ★

GPS TRAILHEAD COORDINATES: N34° 21.131' W85° 40.580'

DISTANCE & CONFIGURATION: 1-mile round-trip

HIKING TIME: 40 minutes

HIGHLIGHTS: Grand waterfalls and swimming holes, abundant wildflowers, dramatic overlooks of the Grand Canyon of the East

ELEVATION: 1,188' at the trailhead, 760' at the river

ACCESS: The preserve is open during daylight hours; no fees. The Little River Canyon Center, home to National Park Service rangers and the Jacksonville State University Field School, is open daily, 10 a.m.–4 p.m. (closed holidays).

MAPS: USGS *Little River*; free NPS maps at the Canyon Center and Little River Falls

FACILITIES: Restrooms at the Canyon Center, Little River Falls, and Eberhart Point; benches along the trail; picnic tables; informational kiosks at all entry points; detailed interpretive information

WHEELCHAIR ACCESS: Possible on the boardwalk to Little River Falls

COMMENTS: Some navigation systems have trouble locating the preserve because of its relatively new street address: 4322 Little River Trail NE, Fort Payne, AL 35967. For now, the old address is more accurate for GPS purposes: 472 Alabama Highway 35, Fort Payne, AL 35967. If you still have trouble finding the preserve, call the number below for directions.

CONTACT: Little River Canyon National Preserve, 256-845-9605, **nps.gov/littlerivercanyon**

Overview

You'll find yourself wondering, *Am I really in Alabama?* Over the course of millions of years, Little River has cut a spectacular gorge in the plateau of Lookout Mountain, leaving exposed sandstone bluffs at the top, a sheltering forest on steep sides, and a river far below that drops off a series of waterfalls and snakes through boulder-strewn rapids and quiet pools.

Route Details

The suggested hike is a steep descent into the canyon from the trailhead at Eberhart Point Overlook, on the canyon road. But before I describe this hike, I'll describe the highlights of getting to the trailhead, because that's at least half of what makes the trip special.

Little River Canyon was designated a national preserve in 1992, which gives it some of the protections afforded to national parks while still allowing hunting and other human activities. Fortunately, it is cared for and curated by the National Park Service, an agency that knows how to host visitors. Little River Canyon has benefited from that. It has also benefited from a partnership with Jacksonville State University, which built the Little River Canyon Center, which serves as both the park headquarters and as an outpost for JSU's environmental-education program.

So that's your first stop, the Canyon Center. Opened in 2009, it's a lovely LEED-certified building with geothermal heating and cooling. A large-screen movie theater shows an orientation film. We found the ranger at the center to be well informed and helpful with maps and directions.

Leaving the center, stop at the parking lot for Little River Falls, just east of the center on AL 35, across the river bridge. We were greeted there by a friendly volunteer ranger. He produced booklets for the kids with quizzes and scavenger hunts to help them find out more about the preserve. The parking area has restrooms (though no running water) and picnic areas with tables and grills.

Little River Canyon National Preserve: Eberhart Trail

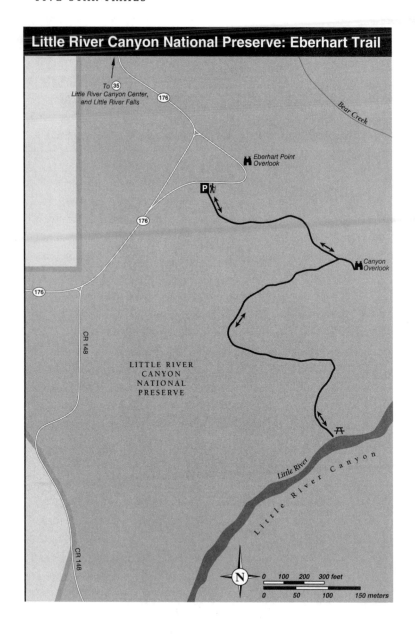

To (35)
Little River Canyon Center,
and Little River Falls

176

Bear Creek

Eberhart Point
Overlook

P

176

176

Canyon
Overlook

CR 148

LITTLE RIVER
CANYON
NATIONAL
PRESERVE

Little River

Little River Canyon

CR 148

N

0   100   200   300 feet

0   50   100   150 meters

A short, extremely well-built, wheelchair-accessible boardwalk leads down to a great overlook of the 45-foot Little River Falls. On one, visit we found water crashing down from almost the full expanse of the falls and throwing up a mist in the process. On a subsequent visit in autumn, the falls were narrower and less dramatic but still impressive. When water is low, some people make their way down to the foot of falls and swim there.

Leaving from that parking lot is a trail down to Martha's Falls, a smaller set of falls downriver. If you're in the mood, this half-mile hike isn't too taxing, though it involves some minor climbing in some steep areas. If you take this trail, avoid the several makeshift spur trails that go straight down to the river. Where the real trail meets the river, there is a broad expanse of rock for sunning and waterfall-gazing. Along this stretch are several traditional swimming spots. Before you think about swimming, though, know that the Little River is not to be trifled with. Water levels vary. When it's wet, the river can be a raging torrent—fun to look at, bad to swim in. When it's dry, extra caution is needed to gauge depth if you're jumping from rocks.

At this point, you've seen only the very tip-top of the canyon. To get a real sense of it, you need to drive the scenic road that traces the western rim. AL 176 is extremely curvy, and you wouldn't want to drop off the edge into the canyon, which deepens dramatically as

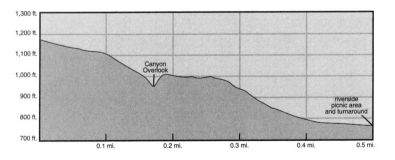

the river tumbles downstream, reaching depths of 500 feet from the rim. To get to the rim road, take a left out of the falls parking lot, recross the river, and take your first left.

Multiple pulloff parking areas along the route offer dramatic overlooks. In addition to the thrill of looking down from the edge, these rugged, rocky overlooks support patches of colorful wildflowers and stunted Virginia pines growing out the shallow pockets of moist soil in the rocks.

The flowers bloom in volume along the roadside in late summer, and the area is one of the best places in the state to see the leaves turn in the fall.

You'll also find a large, distinctive rock in the road, Mushroom Rock. It's a landmark that was saved by the crews assigned to build the road. They disobeyed instructions to knock it down and instead built the road around it. The boulders adjacent to Mushroom Rock offer a place for beginners to play around with rock climbing.

Eberhart Point is just over 11 miles into the scenic drive. You'll find parking areas, restrooms, picnic tables, grills, and an information kiosk. A short, steep, concrete-paved trail leads out to Eberhart Point, if you want to get a view from the top before or after you hike down to the bottom. Looking upstream, generally north, you're looking at the conjunction of two canyons, the main canyon formed by Little River and another coming in from the west, formed by Bear Creek.

For the hike, find the trailhead for Eberhart Trail. It's to the right if you're facing the descent to Eberhart Point. The trail sets off downhill into the woods and shortly joins a wider gravel path that descends steeply to the canyon floor. The trail is only about 0.5 mile long and very steep, but not challenging in a technical sense. It will take some patient exertion to come back up. At the first major switchback, a short path heads to a rocky overlook. It's a great place to look out from, but be careful: It's a steep dropoff.

Returning to the trail and continuing your descent, enjoy the abundant oakleaf hydrangeas, ferns, and rhododendrons that line the trail. Reaching the canyon floor, the trail leads to pebbly shoals on the banks of the river. Along the way you'll notice concrete pillars and the remnants of an old rock building. The area used to be Canyonland Park, which offered a chairlift ride down to a recreation and concession area.

Standing by the riverside and looking up at the surrounding cliffs, you feel a sense of enclosed security instead of the thrill of danger you experience at the rim. Both views inspire awe at the persistence of these tumbling waters. How many millions of years did it take to cut this canyon, to create this jumble of boulders the size of houses?

Just upstream from that beach, we waded up to a set of those boulders that offered a nice place to sun and swim. As stated before, the river varies in its level and force, creating potential dangers if it's too high or too low. If you choose to swim, take care.

Rough, undeveloped trails on the river lead up and down the canyon, but if you do any exploring, keep your eye on the time—you need to be out of the canyon by sunset, and the way you came down is the only way up. And remember that the hike back up is strenuous.

Nearby Attractions

See page 264 for attractions in the Lookout Mountain area.

Directions

Take I-59 North to Exit 218 (Fort Payne/Rainsville). Take a right at the bottom of the ramp and follow AL 35 into Fort Payne. Follow AL 35 left through downtown, then right and up the mountain, following the signs for Little River Canyon. After you make that turn and climb the mountain, it's 7.2 miles to the driveway of the Little River Canyon Center. Stop there to learn about the canyon.

To get to Little River Falls and Martha's Falls, continue from the Canyon Center on AL 35 across the Little River. Parking is on your left. To drive the rim road to Eberhart Point and Trail, take AL 176, which is on the west side of the river, 11.5 miles to the trailhead. Heading back to Birmingham, you can retrace your steps or take AL 176 to Dogtown. From there, take CR 81 to US 11.

Palisades Park & the Bridges of Blount County

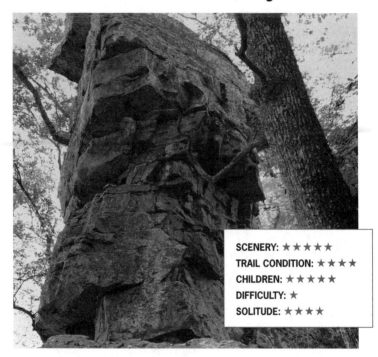

SCENERY: ★ ★ ★ ★ ★
TRAIL CONDITION: ★ ★ ★ ★
CHILDREN: ★ ★ ★ ★ ★
DIFFICULTY: ★
SOLITUDE: ★ ★ ★ ★

GPS TRAILHEAD COORDINATES: N33° 59.301' W86° 27.463'

DISTANCE & CONFIGURATION: 0.5-mile loop

HIKING TIME: 30 minutes

HIGHLIGHTS: Panoramic views from the rocky bluffs of Palisades Park, picnic areas, a playground, and pioneer buildings; cliffs and rock formations that draw crowds for rock climbing and rappelling; three recently restored historic covered bridges; potential for recreation on the beautiful Locust Fork River and its tributaries

ELEVATION: 1,300' atop the bluff, 1,141' at the base of the cliffs

ACCESS: Palisades Park is open January–March, daily, 9 a.m.–5 p.m. April–December, the park stays open until 9 p.m.

MAPS: Available at the park office; map of the Covered Bridge Trail at **tinyurl.com/covered bridgetrail**

FACILITIES: Picnic tables, barbecue grills, pavilions and gazebos, restrooms, playground

WHEELCHAIR ACCESS: Although the hike down the cliffs is not accessible, there are plenty of sights to enjoy in the park atop the bluff.

COMMENTS: Mind your children and yourself around the edges of the bluff at Palisades Park. Sadly, there has already been some vandalism at the newly restored bridges, and trash is a problem, particularly at the Swann Bridge site. Help keep it clean.

CONTACT: 205-274-0017, **blountcountypark.com**

Overview

This trip includes a hike at Palisades Park and a driving circuit of three covered bridges located relatively close together in Blount County. These bridges are not only historic but also feats of nature and works of art. Horton Mill Bridge and Swann Bridge also offer a chance to see beautiful stretches of the Black Warrior River's Locust Fork.

Palisades Park, just outside Oneonta, is worth a visit in and of itself. An 80-acre public park on the bluff of 1,300-foot-tall Ebell Mountain, it contains a quarter-mile of sandstone cliffs 60–70 feet high, atop a bluff overlooking a wide valley. This is a great journey for catching the changing leaves in the fall. The trail at base of the cliffs passes through a profusion of oakleaf hydrangea under the shadows of the grand rock formations.

Route Details

Depending on how you want to shape your day, you have several options on this jaunt. You can head up AL 75 from Birmingham, pass through Oneonta, and see the Horton Mill Covered Bridge before driving across it on your way to Palisades Park. Leaving Palisades Park, you can hit the Easley and Swann Covered Bridges before returning to Birmingham on AL 79. Or you can take the loop in reverse.

Horton Mill Bridge is just off AL 75, north of Oneonta. Look for a small gravel parking lot on the left side of the road (if you're going north). Park in the lot and take in the bridge. Built in 1934, Horton Mill is the tallest historic covered bridge in the United States, crossing 75 feet in the air above the Calvert Prong of the Locust Fork River. It's 220 feet long and has a load limit of 3 tons (if you plan to drive across).

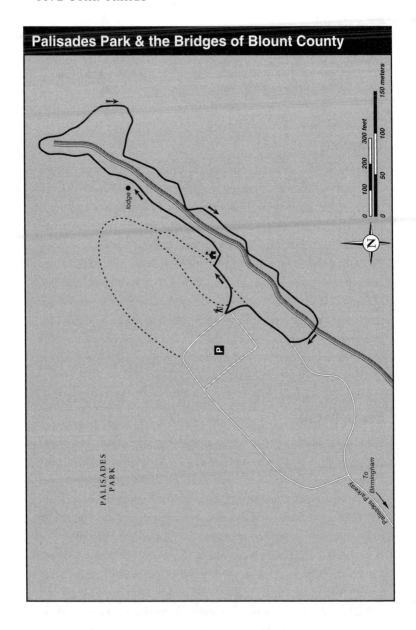

Palisades Park & the Bridges of Blount County

A short trail heads down to the river. It's worth the trip. From that vantage point, you can marvel at the height of the bridge and wonder how they built it. You can also admire the tremendous boulders that fall away from the creek bank. There is a sand beach here, and the river bends and pools around rock formations.

Driving across the one-lane bridge might make you a little nervous, but it's a thrill. Once across, turn right onto Horton Mill Road. Drive 2.5 miles, be alert for a left turn onto on Ebell Road, and look for signs pointing to Palisades Park. A mile later, you take another left onto Palisades Parkway, which leads up to the park.

Stop in at the park office to get a trail map. I chose to do a simple half-mile loop that descends at the northeastern end of the cliffs and walks along their base before climbing back up a gap in the rocks to the south.

This trail route starts on the bluff side of the park office and heads northeast, paralleling the edge of the cliff. Several overlooks along the way are worth a visit.

Follow the trail past a lodge. As the cliffs taper off in height, the trail curves right and downhill, toward the base of the cliffs. As you descend, you'll be amazed at how thick and bountiful the hydrangeas grow all along the mountain slope.

The trail is well worn, though in some stretches it becomes indistinct as it crosses over rocky terrain, but you need not worry about

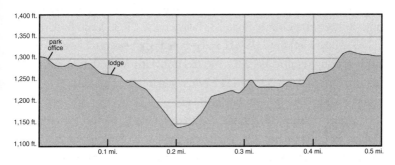

getting lost; just continue along the base of the cliffs. These rock formations are a sight to behold—great tippling, cocked boulders with clefts
in the sandstone formed by the expansion and contraction of the rock
over time. Cracked and fissured, worn and weathered, these cliffs create vertical mazes for rock climbers. If you visit on a weekend, you're
likely to see groups in harnesses climbing and descending.

To get back up to the bluff, you can do a little rock climbing
of your own. You'll find a couple of routes that are options. But if
you continue following the trail to the southwest, the paths become
much easier to mount, as if nature provided a set of stairs for you.

Once back on top, you can walk down farther south on the
bluff to see a decommissioned fire tower. On your way back are more
spots where you can take in the view.

When you're ready to get back on the road, return to Ebell Road
by Palisades Parkway. Take a right, in the direction you came. At the
next intersection, take a left (instead of going right the way you came
in)—this is also Ebell Road. After 1.9 miles, you'll intersect US 231.
Go straight across the road, bearing a little to the left, and pick up
Pine Grove Road. Pine Grove intersects Easley Bridge Road; that road
will be on your right. The Easley Bridge was built in 1927, and like
the other bridges, it has recently been restored with funding from the
Alabama Department of Transportation. It's a shorter bridge, just 95
feet long and not nearly as high as its cousins.

Drive across that bridge and continue on Easley Bridge Road
until it intersects County Road 33. Take a right. CR 33 loops back to
US 231. Take a left onto US 231 and proceed northwest to Cleveland.
After bearing right at US 231's intersection with AL 160, look for a
left turn onto Swann Bridge Road. When you intersect with AL 79, go
straight across onto Swann Bridge Road.

After crossing AL 79, it's less than a mile to Swann Covered
Bridge, which stretches 324 feet across the Locust Fork of the Black
Warrior River. You're asked not to park on the near side of the bridge,
so drive on across, though you should pause to make sure someone
isn't coming from the other direction.

Pulloff parking is available on the far side of the bridge. You can walk down to the river from here and look back to the bridge and up and down the scenic river. Built in 1933, the Swann is the longest covered bridge in Alabama. It's also one of the most beautiful, especially considering its setting.

When you're done, retrace your route back to AL 79 and head south to Birmingham.

Nearby Attractions

If you want to stop for a meal in Oneonta, **Charlie B's Restaurant** serves a classic Southern lunch buffet daily, 11 a.m.–2 p.m. Breakfast is served Saturday, 7–11 a.m. 300 Sixth St. S.; 205-274-7427, **charliebs restaurant.com.**

Legendary bouldering and bluegrass destination **Horse Pens 40** is also in this neck of the woods, just off US 231 between Oneonta and I-59. Horse Pens is a privately owned park on the bluff of Chandler Mountain with great views, hiking trails, and a famous collection of sandstone formations that are also a regional draw for rock climbers. If you want to make it a weekend in Blount County, you can also pay to camp overnight here. For more information, go to **horsepens40.tripod.com.**

Directions

Palisades Park is located at 1225 Palisades Pkwy., just outside Oneonta. Directions for the route to the covered bridges and the park are at the beginning the hike narrative. An interstate alternative is to take I-59 North to Exit 166 (US 231) and go north toward Oneonta. For Palisades Park, continue on US 231 through Oneonta and make a right onto Ebell Road. It's about an hour's drive from Birmingham, either on the interstate or up AL 75.

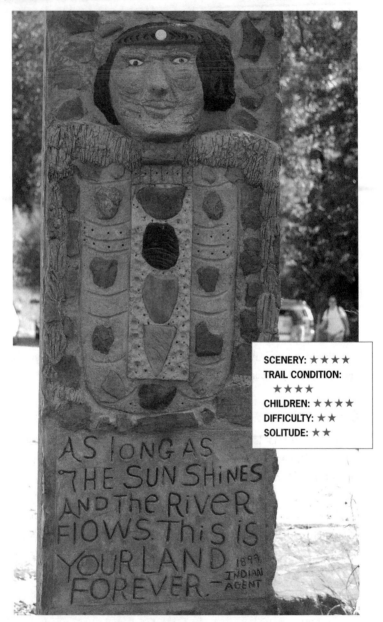

SCENERY: ★ ★ ★ ★
TRAIL CONDITION:
★ ★ ★ ★
CHILDREN: ★ ★ ★ ★
DIFFICULTY: ★ ★
SOLITUDE: ★ ★

AS lONG AS
THE SUN SHiNES
AND THE RiVER
FlOWS. This iS
YOUR LAND 1899
FOREVER. —INDIAN AGENT

GPS TRAILHEAD COORDINATES: N33° 42.176' W86° 41.775'

DISTANCE & CONFIGURATION: 2.3-mile loop

HIKING TIME: 1 hour and 15 minutes

HIGHLIGHTS: Turkey Creek and its falls for fishing, swimming, and sliding; a native-plant eco-scape; highlights of history, ecology, and geology

ELEVATION: 564' above sea level at the trailhead, 800' at the peak of the climb

ACCESS: Hours change seasonally; check the website below for the current schedule. Entrance gates are closed 30 minutes before posted closing time.

MAPS: USGS *Pinson;* a nice trail map is available at **turkeycreeknp.wordpress.com /trail-map.**

FACILITIES: Picnic tables, portable restrooms, information kiosk

WHEELCHAIR ACCESS: None

COMMENTS: Turkey Creek is popular as a swimming hole, but it should be noted that the currents can be swift and the rocks extremely slippery.

CONTACT: Charles Yeager, 205-680-4116, **cyeager@bsc.edu; turkeycreeknp .wordpress.com**

Overview

Covering 466 acres in northeast Jefferson County, the Turkey Creek Nature Preserve has it all: some of the earliest settlement history, the most complex geology, and the most varied ecology you'll find around Birmingham. What's under the water also inspires wonder. Turkey Creek and its tributaries are home to three endangered species of fish, including the vermilion darter, a 2-inch rainbow of a fish that occurs in Turkey Creek and nowhere else in the world. This hike climbs and traverses a ridge above Turkey Creek, then follows a drainage back to scenic Turkey Creek Falls, the preserve's central attraction.

Route Details

There's a fine little loop hike here at the Turkey Creek Nature Preserve, which, according to the preserve's mapping, follows Thompson Trace for 1.4 miles, then returns on Hanby Hollow Trail for 0.9 mile. I measured the route as being a bit shorter. Regardless, it's a pleasant hike that begins with a climb, then follows the ridge before picking up the Hanby Hollow Trail back to Turkey Creek Falls.

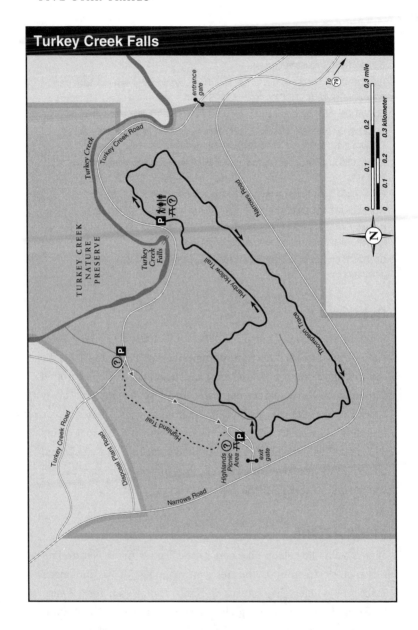

Turkey Creek Falls

It's fitting to start and end at the falls. John Hanby, a veteran of the Creek Indian War of 1813–14, settled here in 1819, the year Alabama became a state. He and his family harnessed the power of the creek by building a mill at Turkey Creek Falls. The family also launched a coal-mining operation and a forge, an early start to Jefferson County's industrial heritage. Those operations prospered until 1865, when, according to local history, Hanby's son, David, was killed by Union soldiers as they swept through Jefferson and Shelby Counties, destroying any industrial operations that supplied the Confederate army.

Though its role as an industrial center ended, Turkey Creek and its falls remained a destination for generations, hosting everything from full-immersion baptism and swimming to raucous late-night partying. Then, in the late 1990s, came a proposal to build a new $50 million county jail on the site. The protest movement that proposal sparked eventually led to the creation of the preserve, now a partnership among Alabama's Forever Wild program, the Freshwater Land Trust, the city of Pinson, and the Southern Environmental Center at Birmingham-Southern College.

I'd like to think that the rejection of the jail proposal was one of those teachable moments that revealed the benefits of working together across community lines and appreciating our natural and cultural assets.

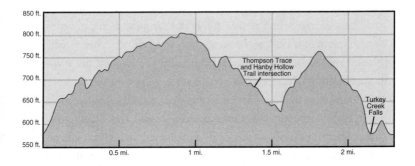

Looking back, the jail proposal seems ridiculous, considering what would have been lost. You've heard of an outdoor classroom? Turkey Creek is an outdoor multidisciplinary college. This little preserve straddles the border of two eco-regions and is a collision point between the limestone-based Valley and Ridge region and the shale hills of the Warrior Coal Field. Four forest types are represented here: the Southeastern Interior Longleaf Pine Woodland, the Allegheny-Cumberland Dry Oak Forest and Woodland, the Cumberland Seepage Forest, and the South Central Interior Small Stream and Riparian Forest.

A tributary of the Black Warrior River, Turkey Creek and its feeder streams support three endangered fish species: the watercress darter (*Etheostoma nuchale*), the rush darter (*Etheostoma phytophilum*), and the vermilion darter (*Etheostoma chermocki*). This information and much more is available at **trekbirmingham.com.**

Without further ado: the hike. The trail leaves from the Turkey Creek Falls parking area, on the left side of the road opposite the creek. The road through the preserve is narrow and one-way. The Thompson Trace Trailhead is on the left side of the parking lot, heading uphill away from the creek.

In the first half-mile, you gain about 130 feet in elevation, enough to get the blood pumping. At the higher elevations, you'll notice longleaf pine, which would be more predominant on these ridges if natural wildfires were more common. Turkey Creek offers a quick getaway from the city, but particularly up here on this ridge, you'll be well aware that civilization is not far away. You can hear a steady stream of traffic on Narrows Road, which is down below. Still, this is a nice walk in the woods. Eventually, the longleaf gives way to an oak-dominated forest as you traverse a draw and drainage. It was around here that our party started noticing double-trunk, triple-trunk, and even quadruple-trunk oak trees. I asked Trek Birmingham author Scot Duncan about this, and he explained that it was evidence that the trees had been cut at some point and the stumps had regenerated multiple sprouts.

At a little over a mile, Thompson Trace intersects the Hanby Hollow Trail. Follow Hanby Hollow downhill, back toward Turkey Creek. Along a small feeder creek, you pass through a glade of ferns and oakleaf hydrangeas. Before you know it, you're back at the parking lot. Cross the street toward the falls, then amble through the ecoscape built as part of Birmingham-Southern's restoration of the area. Where there once was a muddy roadside parking lot, there is now a terraced set of native-plant gardens, permeably surfaced walkways, and other features that capture and retain runoff, allowing it to soak in before entering the creek.

The falls themselves are the central draw. When the water level is right, you can slide down the cold, gushing chute of water into the deep pool below. Large boulders offer opportunities for sunning, observation, and contemplation. You'll often see fly-fisherman downstream. Although we often seek these natural retreats to get away from civilization, you'll usually share the sights of Turkey Creek Falls with someone else. And I, for one, appreciate that. It's a sign that throughout time and despite our different walks in life, we all share an attraction to beautiful places.

Directions

From Birmingham, take Exit 128 off I-20/I-59 and head north on AL 79 (Tallapoosa Street). Continue on AL 79 for almost 12 miles. At the intersection of AL 79 and AL 75, turn left onto Narrows Road. After 0.2 mile, turn right onto Turkey Creek Road. The gravel parking lot for the falls is on the left about half a mile after that turn, opposite the creek.

Appendix A: Suggested Reading & Reference

Books

Duncan, R. Scot. *Southern Wonder: Alabama's Surprising Biodiversity*. Tuscaloosa: University of Alabama Press, 2013.

Finch, Bill, and Beth Maynor Young. *Longleaf, Far as the Eye Can See: A New Vision of North America's Richest Forest*. Chapel Hill: University of North Carolina Press, 2012.

Lacefield, Jim. *Lost Worlds in Alabama Rocks: A Guide to the State's Ancient Life and Landscapes*. 2nd ed. Tuscaloosa: Alabama Museum of Natural History, 2013.

White, Marjorie Longenecker. *The Birmingham District: An Industrial History and Guide*. Birmingham: Birmingham Historical Society, 1981. (See **bhistorical.org /publications** for additional BHS books.)

Young, Beth Maynor, and John C. Hall. *Headwaters: A Journey on Alabama Rivers*. Tuscaloosa: University of Alabama Press, 2009.

Websites

ALABAMA BIRDING TRAILS
alabamabirdingtrails.com
Statewide network of prime bird-watching locations.

ALABAMA STATE PARKS
alapark.com
Information on Oak Mountain and Cheaha State Parks, which are featured in this book, as well as other state parks like Lake Guntersville, Buck's Pocket, and DeSoto.

BHAMWIKI
bhamwiki.com
A locally maintained wiki focused on Birmingham, from history to current events.

BIRMINGHAM RAILS
bhamrails.info
Industrial and railroad history of the Birmingham area.

NATIONAL FORESTS IN ALABAMA
www.fs.usda.gov/alabama
Information on the Talladega District of the Talladega National Forest, which contains the Cheaha Wilderness Area, and on the Bankhead National Forest, which contains the Sipsey Wilderness Area.

NATIONAL WILDLIFE REFUGES IN ALABAMA
fws.gov/refuges/refugelocatormaps/alabama.html
Information on Cahaba River, Wheeler, and other National Wildlife Refuges.

ONLINE ENCYCLOPEDIA OF ALABAMA
encyclopediaofalabama.org
Reliably sourced information on history, geography, and a little of everything else.

OUTDOOR ALABAMA
outdooralabama.com
Official website of the Alabama Department of Conservation and Natural Resources.

OUTSIDE ALABAMA
outsidealabama.com
Statewide online publication focused on outdoor pursuits.

PINHOTI TRAIL ALLIANCE
pinhotitrailalliance.org
If you're going hiking on the Pinhoti, get information here.

ROOTSRATED
rootsrated.com/birmingham-al
A locally sourced directory of outdoor recreational opportunities.

TREK BIRMINGHAM
trekbirmingham.com
An educational and recreational resource guide for the Greater Birmingham area, provided by Birmingham-Southern College's Urban Environmental Studies Program.

Appendix B:
Outdoor Retailers

ACADEMY SPORTS + OUTDOORS
academy.com

310 Doug Baker Blvd.
Birmingham, AL 35242
205-981-4150

2810 John Hawkins Pkwy.
Hoover, AL 35244
205-403-6145

1612 Gadsden Hwy.
Trussville, AL 35235
205-661-1140

ALABAMA OUTDOORS
alabamaoutdoors.com

3054 Independence Dr.
Homewood, AL 35209
205-870-1919

4710 Frank St., #116
Trussville, AL 35235
205-655-6025

108 Inverness Plaza
Birmingham, AL 35242
205-980-3303

DICK'S SPORTING GOODS
dickssportinggoods.com

5201 US Hwy. 280
Birmingham, AL 35242
205-981-1320

4401 Creekside Ave.
Hoover, AL 35244
205-909-1400

MARK'S OUTDOOR SPORTS
marksoutdoors.com

1400 Montgomery Hwy.
Vestavia Hills, AL 35216
205-822-2010

MOUNTAIN HIGH OUTFITTERS
mountainhighoutfitters.com

2800 Cahaba Village Plaza, #250
Birmingham, AL 35243
205-970-3300

1901 Sixth Ave. N., #299
Birmingham, AL 35203
205-321-6562

127 Summit Blvd.
Birmingham, AL 35243
205-967-7607

2000-147A Riverchase Galleria
Hoover, AL 35244
205-985-3215

ROGERS TRADING COMPANY
facebook.com/rogerstradingco

140 Resource Center Pkwy.
Birmingham, AL 35242
205-408-9378

SIMMONS SPORTING GOODS
simmonssportinggoods.net

2001 Second Ave. N.
Bessemer, AL 35020
205-425-4720

Appendix C:
Hiking & Outdoor Clubs

BIRMINGHAM ADVENTURE GROUP
meetup.com/birminghamadventuregroup
Connect with other local outdoor-adventure enthusiasts through this Meetup group. Hiking, kayaking, canoeing, backpacking, camping, and other outdoor excursions.

BIRMINGHAM URBAN MOUNTAIN PEDALERS
800-960-9457, **bump.org**
A recreation and service group for Birmingham-area mountain biking enthusiasts.

FRESH AIR FAMILY
205-540-6642, **freshairfamily.org**
Outdoor adventures and education geared to families with children.

SOUTHEASTERN OUTINGS
seoutings.blogspot.com
A nonprofit organization that sponsors simple outdoor adventures. All activities are open to the public.

UAB ADVENTURE EDUCATION PROGRAM
uab.edu/campusrecreation/adventure-rec-home
Offers a series of organized outings; provides an extensive selection of equipment for rent to the public for camping, boating, and biking.

Appendix D: Advocacy & Volunteer Groups

ALABAMA FOREVER WILD LAND TRUST
alabamaforeverwild.com

A program of the Alabama Department of Conservation & Natural Resources, this land-preservation project protects ecologically and recreationally important lands. The interactive website lets you explore properties and get information and directions.

ALABAMA HIKING TRAIL SOCIETY
256-786-0894, **hikealabama.org**

Advocacy for and support and maintenance of trails statewide. Local chapters include one in Birmingham.

FRESHWATER LAND TRUST
freshwaterlandtrust.org

Develops and maintains open spaces that protect rivers, streams, and endangered freshwater species throughout Alabama. See page 295 for more information.

THE FRIENDS OF RED MOUNTAIN PARK
friendsofredmountainpark.org

Volunteer organization dedicated to trail building, improvements, and guided hikes at Red Mountain Park. See the last page of this book for more information.

VULCAN TRAIL ASSOCIATION
vulcantrailassociation.ws

Founded in 1977, the VTA promotes hiking and is also involved in trail maintenance. Organizes group backpacking, rafting, canoeing, and biking trips. Meets the third Wednesday of every month (except July, November, and December) at 7 p.m. at the Hoover Public Library: 205-444-7800, **hooverlibrary.org.**

Index

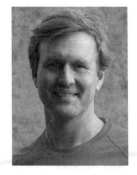

Born in Birmingham, **THOMAS SPENCER** grew up hiking and camping in his native state, and for two decades he crisscrossed Alabama as a reporter for *The Anniston Star* and *The Birmingham News,* specializing in coverage of the outdoors and the environment. During his reporting career, he covered the acquisition of the Walls of Jericho, the protection of endangered species, the development of recreational assets such as the Alabama Scenic River Trail and the Pinhoti Trail, and the movement to expand green space and trails in the Birmingham metro area. A graduate of the University of Virginia, Tom is now the senior research associate at the Public Affairs Research Council of Alabama, based at Samford University. An Eagle Scout, he is a founder of The Friends of Red Mountain Park and serves on the board of the Cahaba River Society.

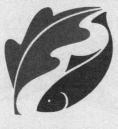

FRESHWATER
LAND TRUST

The Freshwater Land Trust is a nonprofit organization whose mission is the acquisition and stewardship of lands that enhance water quality and preserve open space. Since 1996, we have worked to acquire, conserve, and connect open spaces that are critical for the protection of rivers and streams and that provide recreational opportunities for the community. The Freshwater Land Trust owns and manages more than 5,000 acres in Jefferson County, making it one of the largest owners of private nature preserves in the state of Alabama. With our partners, we have helped protect over 10,000 acres.

Our organization takes a practical approach to conservation and focuses on building partnerships with the public, private, and government sectors. We work to ensure that everyone wins: landowners, businesses, and communities alike. Our projects include Red Mountain Park, the Five Mile Creek Greenway Partnership, the Red Rock Ridge and Valley Trail System, Turkey Creek Nature Preserve, Tapawingo Springs, Moss Rock Preserve expansion, Wildwood Preserve in Homewood, Homewood Forest Preserve, and the Cahaba Riverwalk on Grants Mill Road.

The Freshwater Land Trust was the first nationally accredited land trust in Alabama, through the Land Trust Accreditation Commission. Based in Birmingham, FWLT is committed to preserving the places that matter in Bibb, Blount, Chilton, Jefferson, Shelby, St. Clair, and Walker Counties. In the past 17 years, not only have we preserved land and enhanced water quality, but we've protected habitats that are critical to endangered freshwater species—many of which are found only in Alabama. These successes have also greatly increased the quality of life for the citizens of our communities by providing additional recreational opportunities.

To find out more, visit **freshwaterlandtrust.org.**

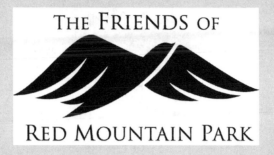

THE FRIENDS OF

RED MOUNTAIN PARK

The Friends of Red Mountain Park is a group of volunteers who are united in thinking that Red Mountain Park will be a win–win situation for all of us in Birmingham. We are a 501(c)(3) nonprofit organization that serves as a bridge between the community and the park's commission and staff. Throughout the planning process, we have striven to bring all interested voices to the table and give everyone a way to participate in this great project.

Our goals are to spread the word about this project, volunteer our time and talent to enhance the park's development, and champion the use and enjoyment of the park for the broadest range of citizens. To become a Friend of Red Mountain Park or to contribute, visit **friends ofredmountainpark.org.**

About Red Mountain Park

Red Mountain Park's 1,300-acre wooded site is located in Birmingham, 3 miles west of I-65 (Exit 255, Lakeshore Parkway). Visitors enjoy 11 miles of walking, hiking and mountain biking trails; the Red Ore Zip Tour, a 1½-hour zip line adventure through the trees; the Hugh Kaul Beanstalk Forest, a treetop course with 20 unique rope and cable challenges; and Remy's Dog Park, a 6-acre off-leash dog retreat. Beautiful destination sites—the historic Redding Hoist House, three treehouse views (SkyHy Treehouse, Riley's Roost Treehouse, and Rushing Rendezvous Treehouse), and glimpses of iron ore mine entrances—both surprise and delight our guests. Upon completion of Phase 2 Development in 2016, the park will deliver even more trails, picnic pavilions and an event facility, formal entry and parking, and an adventure-activity center.

For more information, visit **redmountainpark.org.**